The 15-Minute Flat Belly Fix

Rapid Ab Workouts to Burn Belly Fat and Sculpt Your Core

SAM ERIC

DEDICATION

To my family, whose unwavering support and love have been my foundation,

To my friends, who have inspired and encouraged me every step of the way,

And to all the dreamers and doers, who strive for success and never give up,

This book is dedicated to you.

May it be a guide and a source of inspiration on your journey to achieving your dreams.

With heartfelt gratitude.

Abstract

The 15-Minute Flat Belly Fix: Rapid Ab Workouts to Burn Belly Fat and Sculpt Your Core is a comprehensive fitness guide designed for individuals seeking quick, efficient, and impactful routines to reduce belly fat, strengthen their core, and enhance overall body composition. This book provides a series of high-intensity, time-efficient workouts specifically tailored to target the abdominal muscles, including both the upper and lower abs, obliques, and deep core stabilizers. Each workout is carefully structured to deliver maximum fat-burning results in just 15 minutes per session, making it ideal for busy individuals who want to achieve a flat, toned belly without spending hours in the gym.

The book outlines an easy-to-follow 15-minute daily routine that combines strength-building exercises with high-intensity interval training (HIIT) to elevate metabolism, accelerate fat loss, and sculpt the core. With an emphasis on core engagement and proper form, the routines are designed to ensure that readers maximize the effectiveness of each movement while minimizing the risk of injury. Additionally, the book incorporates tips on incorporating cardio for enhanced calorie burn and interval-based exercises for a dynamic approach to fat loss.

Beyond the workouts, *The 15-Minute Flat Belly Fix* also offers expert nutrition tips and strategies for flattening the belly, emphasizing the role of clean eating, hydration, and gut health. The book provides a practical, sustainable approach to nutrition that complements the workouts and promotes fat-burning foods, like lean proteins, healthy fats, and high-fiber vegetables.

The book's user-friendly format includes detailed instructions, visual aids, and customizable workout plans, making it accessible to people of all fitness levels, from beginners to advanced exercisers. Whether the goal is to trim down belly fat, tone the core, or simply improve overall health, this book equips readers with the tools and knowledge needed to transform their midsection, boost their confidence, and achieve lasting results in minimal time.

In summary, *The 15-Minute Flat Belly Fix* is an essential resource for anyone looking to enhance their fitness routine, achieve a leaner, stronger core, and boost overall body strength, all while fitting into a busy schedule. With its straightforward approach, this book empowers readers to take control of their fitness journey and achieve a flat, sculpted belly without the need for hours of intense training.

Introduction: Welcome to the 15-Minute Flat Belly Fix

The modern world moves fast, and for most of us, time is a luxury. Between work commitments, family responsibilities, and personal obligations, carving out hours for the gym or cooking elaborate meals often feels impossible. Yet, health and fitness remain non-negotiable priorities for living a vibrant, confident, and energetic life. That's where this book, The 15-Minute Flat Belly Fix, comes in.

This isn't just another fitness guide; it's your ultimate roadmap to achieving a toned and strong core while burning stubborn belly fat—all in just 15 minutes a day. Whether you're a busy parent, a working professional, or someone new to fitness, this program fits seamlessly into your schedule without sacrificing effectiveness.

Purpose of the Book

Empower Readers with Quick, Effective Ab Workouts

The primary goal of this book is to show you that fitness doesn't have to be time-consuming to be impactful. In just 15 minutes a day, you can:

- Target your core muscles with precision.
- Build strength, stability, and definition.

- Kickstart fat-burning processes that continue even after your workout ends.

These workouts are designed for everyone—regardless of fitness level. From beginners to seasoned fitness enthusiasts, you'll find exercises that challenge you without overwhelming you.

Emphasize a Holistic Approach

While effective workouts form the backbone of this program, they're only part of the equation. Sustainable results come from addressing every aspect of your health. This book takes a holistic approach, focusing on three critical pillars:

1. **Workouts:** Structured, efficient routines that target belly fat and strengthen your core.
2. **Nutrition:** A straightforward guide to fueling your body with foods that promote fat loss and energy.
3. **Lifestyle Changes:** Practical tips on motivation, stress management, and sleep optimization to support your journey.

By integrating these elements, you'll not only achieve a flatter belly but also enhance your overall well-being.

Why 15 Minutes?

The Science Behind Short, Intense Workouts

You might wonder: can 15 minutes really make a difference? The answer is a resounding yes—and here's why:

1. **High-Intensity Interval Training (HIIT):**
   - Short bursts of intense exercise followed by brief rest periods maximize calorie burn in minimal time.
   - HIIT workouts boost your metabolism and trigger the afterburn effect (Excess Post-Exercise Oxygen Consumption, or EPOC), meaning your body continues burning calories long after you've finished.
2. **Focus on Core Engagement:**
   - A targeted 15-minute session focusing on your core muscles delivers noticeable results by isolating and strengthening key areas.
3. **Time Efficiency Meets Consistency:**
   - When workouts are short and accessible, you're more likely to stick with them, making consistency—one of the most critical factors in fitness—achievable.

Benefits for Core Strengthening and Fat-Burning Efficiency

- **Core Strengthening:** Your core muscles support almost every movement you make, from walking to lifting. Strong core muscles enhance your posture, reduce back pain, and improve overall functionality.
- **Fat-Burning Efficiency:** Belly fat, especially visceral fat, is stubborn and linked to health risks. Short, intense workouts combine cardio and strength elements to target and reduce this fat effectively.
- **Improved Fitness in Less Time:** Research shows that shorter, intense workouts can be just as effective as longer sessions, making them ideal for busy individuals.

By focusing on quality over quantity, the 15-minute format ensures maximum impact with minimum time investment.

Overview of the Program

This book is built around a simple yet effective formula:
15 minutes of focused effort daily = noticeable results over time.

Rapid Ab Workouts

The heart of the program lies in fast-paced, highly effective ab routines designed to:

- Strengthen and sculpt your core.
- Burn calories by incorporating dynamic, fat-burning movements. The workouts are divided into beginner, intermediate, and advanced levels, allowing you to progress at your own pace.

Nutrition Strategies

A flat belly isn't achieved through exercise alone. Nutrition plays a pivotal role, and this program provides you with:

- **Simple, actionable dietary advice:** Learn what to eat, when to eat, and how to avoid common dietary pitfalls.
- **Meal planning tips:** Create quick, nutrient-dense meals that support fat loss without adding stress to your day.
- **Flat-belly-friendly recipes:** Enjoy meals and snacks that are as delicious as they are effective.

Motivation and Consistency Tips

Sticking to a fitness routine requires more than just willpower—it requires a mindset shift. This book offers tools to help you stay motivated, such as:

- **Goal-setting strategies:** Break down long-term aspirations into achievable milestones.

- **Overcoming setbacks:** Learn how to bounce back from plateaus, missed workouts, or dietary slip-ups.
- **Building habits that last:** Incorporate fitness and wellness into your daily life effortlessly.

What to Expect

As you journey through this book, you'll discover:

- A deeper understanding of how your core works and why it's central to overall fitness.
- Workouts that are accessible, adaptable, and energizing.
- Practical advice to improve not just your appearance but your confidence and health.

The 15-Minute Flat Belly Fix is more than a fitness program—it's a lifestyle upgrade that empowers you to look and feel your best, no matter how hectic your schedule gets. Let's get started on the path to a stronger core, a flatter belly, and a healthier you!

Part 1: Understanding the Core and Belly Fat

Chapter 1: Core Anatomy and Function

To achieve a flat belly and sculpted core, it's essential to first understand how your core functions and why it plays such a vital role in your overall health. This chapter dives into the anatomy of your core, the role of each muscle group, and how a strong core benefits more than just your physical appearance.

The Role of Core Muscles

Your core isn't just about your abs—it's a complex system of muscles that work together to stabilize and move your torso. These muscles form a cylindrical powerhouse in the center of your body, and each group plays a unique role:

1. Rectus Abdominis

- Often referred to as the "six-pack," this long, flat muscle runs vertically along the front of your abdomen.
- **Function:**
    - Flexes the spine (e.g., during crunches or sit-ups).

- Helps with bending forward and stabilizing the body during dynamic movements.
- **Importance in a Flat Belly:**
  - The rectus abdominis is what gives the appearance of defined abs when body fat is reduced.

2. Obliques

- Located on the sides of your abdomen, the obliques are divided into two parts: internal and external obliques.
- **Function:**
  - Assist in twisting and bending movements.
  - Help with lateral stability and rotation of the torso.
- **Importance in Everyday Life:**
  - Strengthening the obliques improves movements like turning, reaching, and stabilizing your body during side-to-side motions.

3. Transverse Abdominis (TVA)

- This deep, corset-like muscle wraps around your torso horizontally beneath the rectus abdominis.
- **Function:**
  - Compresses the abdomen, providing stability to the spine and pelvis.

- o Plays a key role in core bracing, essential for maintaining posture and protecting the lower back.
- **Importance for Core Strength:**
  - o A strong TVA is the foundation for all core movements, reducing injury risk and enhancing overall athletic performance.

4. Lower Back Muscles (Erector Spinae and Multifidus)

- These muscles run along the spine and support its natural curves.
- **Function:**
  - o Stabilize the spine during movement.
  - o Work with the abs to maintain an upright posture.
- **Importance in Core Health:**
  - o Weak lower back muscles can lead to poor posture and back pain, making core strengthening a balanced effort.

Why a Strong Core is Essential

A well-conditioned core is about much more than aesthetics; it's integral to how your body moves and functions daily. Here's why a strong core is critical:

1. Core Stability and Balance

- The core is the foundation of all movement. A strong core stabilizes your spine and pelvis, allowing your arms and legs to move freely and effectively.
- **Examples:**
  - Balancing while standing on one foot.
  - Maintaining stability during dynamic activities like running or jumping.

2. Improved Posture

- A weak core often leads to slouching, forward head posture, and lower back pain.
- Strengthening the core helps align your spine, reducing strain on surrounding muscles and joints.
- **Benefits:**
  - A straight posture not only looks confident but also improves breathing and reduces fatigue caused by inefficient movement patterns.

3. Enhanced Athletic Performance

- Many sports and physical activities rely on core strength for power and precision.
- **Examples:**
  - The twisting motion in a tennis swing or golf drive.
  - The explosive power needed for sprinting or jumping.

4. Injury Prevention

- A strong core protects the lower back by providing support during heavy lifting, bending, or sudden movements.
- It also reduces the risk of overcompensation injuries in other areas like the shoulders or hips.

5. Everyday Functionality

- Core strength plays a role in nearly every daily activity, from bending to pick up groceries to reaching for something on a high shelf.
- A stable, strong core ensures these movements are efficient and pain-free.

6. Fat-Burning Benefits

- Engaging the core during workouts activates large muscle groups, increasing calorie burn.
- Dynamic core exercises that combine movement with strength improve metabolism and contribute to overall fat loss.

The Core as Your Body's Powerhouse

Think of your core as the control center of your body. Whether you're standing, sitting, or moving, your core muscles are always working. Developing these muscles not only gives you a toned midsection but also enhances your physical resilience, functional strength, and overall health.

This foundational understanding of core anatomy and function will guide you as you progress through the program. By targeting these key muscles with the right exercises and strategies, you'll unlock the potential of your core to transform not just your physique but your quality of life.

Let's begin by exploring how the right exercises can strengthen and sculpt these muscles in the chapters ahead.

Chapter 2: The Truth About Belly Fat

Achieving a flat belly goes beyond just strengthening your core muscles; it requires a deeper understanding of the types of belly fat, what causes it, and how to effectively reduce it. In this chapter, we'll explore the science behind belly fat, its root causes, and why a combined approach of exercise and nutrition is key to burning fat and sculpting your core.

Types of Belly Fat

Not all belly fat is created equal. Understanding the two main types of belly fat can help you target and reduce it more effectively.

1. Subcutaneous Fat

- **What it is:**
  - Subcutaneous fat is the layer of fat located directly beneath the skin.
  - It's the fat you can pinch with your fingers around your waist or abdomen.
- **Role in the body:**
  - Acts as an energy reserve and provides insulation and cushioning for the body.
- **Health implications:**
  - While subcutaneous fat is less harmful than visceral fat, excessive

amounts can still contribute to health issues and hinder physical performance.

2. Visceral Fat

- **What it is:**
  - o Visceral fat is deeper fat that surrounds internal organs like the liver, pancreas, and intestines.
- **Role in the body:**
  - o A small amount of visceral fat is normal and protects organs, but too much can be dangerous.
- **Health implications:**
  - o Excess visceral fat is associated with serious health risks, including heart disease, type 2 diabetes, and metabolic syndrome.
  - o It also contributes to the classic "beer belly" appearance, which is firm to the touch.

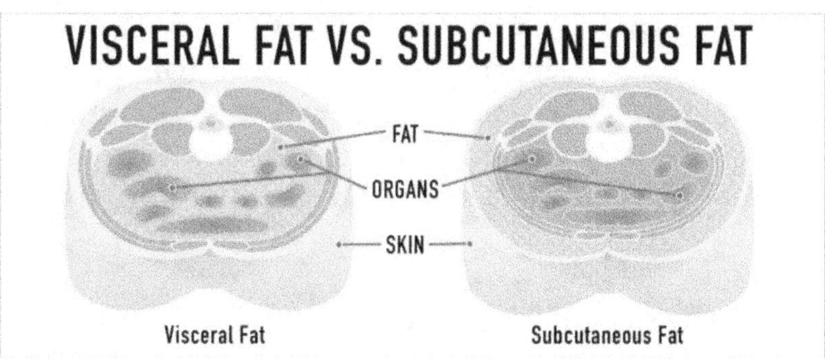

Key Difference Between Subcutaneous and Visceral Fat

- Subcutaneous fat affects appearance and is easier to reduce through diet and exercise.
- Visceral fat poses greater health risks and responds more to lifestyle changes like consistent physical activity and improved nutrition.

Common Causes of Belly Fat

Belly fat doesn't accumulate overnight. It results from a combination of factors, many of which are within your control. Let's examine the most common causes:

1. Poor Diet

- **Excess Calories:** Consuming more calories than you burn leads to fat storage, particularly in the abdominal area.
- **Sugary Foods and Drinks:** Foods high in refined sugars (e.g., sodas, candy, and pastries) spike blood sugar levels, causing insulin resistance and fat storage.
- **Low Protein and Fiber Intake:** Diets lacking in protein and fiber often lead to overeating because these nutrients promote satiety.

2. Sedentary Lifestyle

- Lack of physical activity is one of the primary contributors to weight gain and fat accumulation.
- Sitting for long hours reduces calorie burn and lowers metabolism, making it easier to gain weight in the midsection.
- Without exercise, muscle mass decreases over time, further reducing the body's fat-burning capacity.

3. Stress and Hormonal Imbalances

- **Cortisol and Belly Fat:** Chronic stress triggers the release of cortisol, a hormone that promotes fat storage, especially around the abdomen.
- **Hormonal Changes:** Hormonal shifts during menopause or as a result of conditions like polycystic ovary syndrome (PCOS) can also lead to increased belly fat.
- **Stress Eating:** Emotional stress often leads to overeating, especially of comfort foods high in sugar and fat, which contribute to belly fat.

The Importance of Combining Exercise with Nutrition for Fat Loss

When it comes to reducing belly fat, no single solution works in isolation. A combined approach of exercise and nutrition is essential for effective and sustainable fat loss. Here's why:

1. Exercise Burns Calories and Builds Muscle

- **Calorie Deficit:** Physical activity helps create a calorie deficit, a critical component of fat loss.
- **Muscle Growth:** Strength training (including core exercises) builds lean muscle, which boosts metabolism and increases calorie burn even at rest.
- **Targeted Fat Loss Myth:** While you can't spot-reduce fat in one specific area, engaging in a full-body workout routine helps reduce overall fat, including belly fat.

2. Nutrition Fuels Fat Loss

- **Balanced Diet:** A diet rich in lean protein, healthy fats, and complex carbohydrates provides the nutrients your body needs while promoting fat loss.
- **Portion Control:** Reducing portion sizes and cutting back on processed foods can help manage calorie intake.
- **Reducing Inflammation:** Eating whole, unprocessed foods lowers inflammation, which is linked to belly fat accumulation.

3. The Synergy of Exercise and Nutrition

- **Sustainable Results:** Exercise helps burn fat and improve muscle tone, while a proper diet prevents new fat accumulation.

- **Improved Energy Levels:** Eating well and staying active boosts energy levels, making it easier to stick to your fitness routine.
- **Enhanced Metabolism:** Regular physical activity combined with a nutrient-rich diet keeps your metabolism working efficiently.

Why Understanding Belly Fat Matters

Belly fat is more than a cosmetic concern—it's a health issue that requires attention. By understanding the types of belly fat and what causes it, you can make informed decisions about your diet and exercise routine. The combination of knowledge, action, and consistency will set you on the path to not only achieving a flatter belly but also improving your overall health and vitality.

In the next chapters, we'll dive deeper into the specific exercises, routines, and strategies designed to help you tackle belly fat head-on.

Chapter 3: The Science Behind 15-Minute Workouts

When time is limited, maximizing the efficiency of your workouts becomes crucial. The 15-minute workout approach isn't just convenient—it's rooted in science. This chapter explores why short, intense workouts are highly effective for fat burning, the difference between High-Intensity Interval Training (HIIT) and traditional cardio, and the specific benefits of targeted ab exercises for sculpting and toning your core.

How Short Workouts Can Maximize Fat Burning

The effectiveness of 15-minute workouts lies in their ability to activate your metabolism and burn fat long after the session ends. Here's how it works:

The EPOC Effect (Excess Post-Exercise Oxygen Consumption)

- After intense exercise, your body continues to burn calories as it works to return to its pre-exercise state. This is known as the afterburn effect or EPOC.
- **What happens during EPOC?**
    - Your body replenishes oxygen levels, restores muscle glycogen, and repairs muscle tissue.

- These processes require energy, which means additional calories are burned post-workout.

Why Short, Intense Workouts Trigger EPOC

- Intensity is the key factor. Short bursts of high-intensity exercise elevate your heart rate and push your muscles to their limits, stimulating greater oxygen demand.
- Studies show that high-intensity workouts, even when brief, can result in higher EPOC compared to steady-state exercise like jogging.

Key Fat-Burning Takeaway

You don't need an hour-long gym session to achieve results. A 15-minute, well-structured workout can torch calories during and after your session, making it an efficient option for busy schedules.

High-Intensity Interval Training (HIIT) vs. Traditional Cardio

What is HIIT?

High-Intensity Interval Training (HIIT) involves alternating between short bursts of intense effort and brief recovery periods. For example, sprinting for 30 seconds followed by walking for 30 seconds is a classic HIIT format.

Benefits of HIIT Over Traditional Cardio

1. **Time Efficiency:**
   - HIIT workouts can deliver the same (or better) results in a fraction of the time compared to steady-state cardio.
2. **Enhanced Calorie Burn:**
   - HIIT elevates your heart rate more dramatically, increasing calorie burn during and after exercise.
3. **Improved Fitness Levels:**
   - HIIT combines cardio and strength elements, improving both endurance and muscular strength.
4. **Muscle Preservation:**
   - Traditional cardio can lead to muscle loss if overdone. HIIT, on the other hand, builds and preserves muscle while burning fat.

Drawbacks of Traditional Cardio

- While steady-state cardio (e.g., jogging or cycling) has its benefits, it requires more time to achieve similar results.
- Over-reliance on traditional cardio can lead to a plateau, as your body becomes efficient at the activity and burns fewer calories over time.

Benefits of Targeted Ab Exercises for Sculpting and Toning

Why Targeted Ab Exercises Matter

While overall fat loss is necessary to reveal a toned core, targeted exercises are essential for strengthening and sculpting the muscles underneath.

1. **Improved Muscle Definition:**
   - Ab-focused exercises like planks, crunches, and leg raises build strength and enhance the appearance of your rectus abdominis, obliques, and transverse abdominis.
2. **Enhanced Core Stability:**
   - A strong core improves balance, posture, and overall functionality.
3. **Boosted Fat-Burning Potential:**
   - Engaging your core during dynamic movements activates multiple muscle groups, increasing calorie burn.

Dynamic Ab Exercises and Their Advantages

- Traditional crunches are effective, but incorporating dynamic movements like bicycle crunches, mountain climbers, or Russian twists engages your core more fully, promoting functional strength and fat burning.

Ab Exercises and Functional Fitness

A strong core isn't just about aesthetics. It supports everyday activities like lifting, bending, and twisting, as well as athletic performance.

The Science in Action

The combination of HIIT principles and targeted ab exercises creates a powerful synergy:

- **HIIT burns fat efficiently, including stubborn belly fat.**
- **Ab exercises strengthen and sculpt your core muscles, helping to reveal definition as fat is reduced.**

By integrating these strategies into 15-minute sessions, you can achieve a flat belly faster without sacrificing results. The next chapters will outline specific workouts designed to put this science into practice.

Part 2: The 15-Minute Workout Plan

Chapter 4: Getting Started

Before diving into the workouts, preparation is key. This chapter lays the foundation for success, covering everything you need to get started with the 15-Minute Flat Belly Fix. By ensuring you have the right mindset, equipment, and environment, you'll be ready to maximize the effectiveness of your workouts.

The Minimalist Approach to Fitness

One of the greatest advantages of the 15-Minute Flat Belly Fix is its simplicity. You don't need a gym membership or expensive equipment. In fact, all you need is a small space, a few optional tools, and your own bodyweight.

Essential Equipment

The program is designed to work with minimal gear, making it accessible to everyone. Here's what you might consider having on hand:

1. **Yoga Mat (or Exercise Mat)**
   - **Purpose:** Provides cushioning for your joints and ensures grip during exercises.

- o **Tip:** If you don't have a mat, a carpeted area or folded towel can suffice.

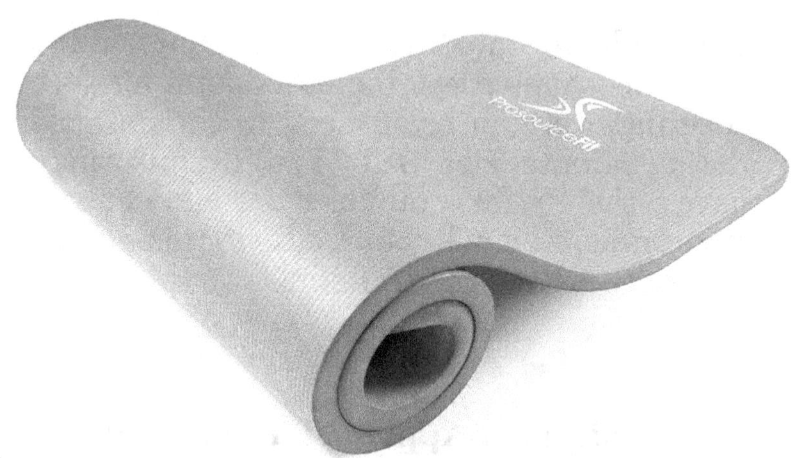

2. **Resistance Bands (Optional)**
   - o **Purpose:** Adds intensity to bodyweight exercises, especially for engaging deeper core muscles.
   - o **Examples:** Use a resistance band for bicycle crunches or seated twists for added challenge.

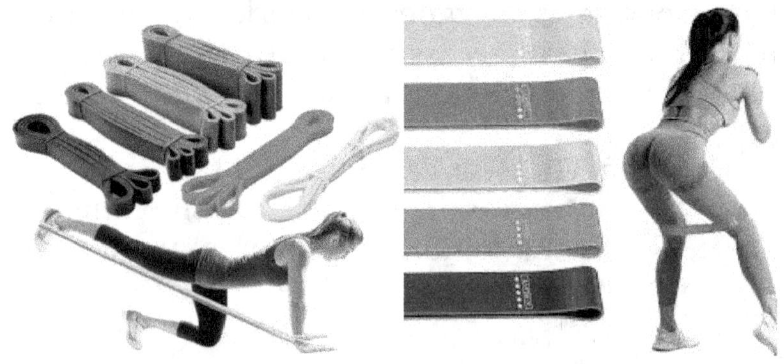

3. **Dumbbells or Kettlebell (Optional)**
   - o **Purpose:** Adds weight to increase muscle engagement and calorie burn.
   - o **Examples:** Holding a light dumbbell during Russian twists or overhead while performing sit-ups increases resistance.
4. **A Chair or Sturdy Surface (Optional)**
   - o **Purpose:** Assists with modifications, such as incline planks or seated leg lifts for beginners.
5. **Water Bottle and Towel**
   - o **Purpose:** Staying hydrated and wiping away sweat ensures comfort during your workout.

Bodyweight: The Ultimate Tool

Even without any equipment, your own bodyweight is enough to sculpt your core and burn fat. Exercises like planks, mountain climbers, and leg raises are highly effective at building strength and definition.

Setting Up Your Workout Space

A small, dedicated space is all you need to complete your 15-minute workouts. Here's how to create an environment that keeps you focused:

1. **Find a Flat Surface:** Ensure there's enough room to lie down, stretch out, and move freely.
2. **Declutter Your Space:** Remove distractions like clutter or unnecessary furniture.
3. **Lighting and Ventilation:** A well-lit, airy room can boost your energy and mood during workouts.
4. **Music or Silence:** Choose a workout playlist to stay motivated, or embrace silence to focus on form and breathing.

Mindset and Preparation

Preparing your body and mind for consistent effort will ensure you stick to the program and see results.

1. Start with a Warm-Up

- Spend 2–3 minutes performing light cardio (e.g., jogging in place or jumping jacks) to increase blood flow and loosen your muscles.
- Add dynamic stretches like arm circles or torso twists to prepare your core for action.

2. Commit to Consistency

- **Remember:** It's only 15 minutes. Block out this time in your day as a non-negotiable appointment with yourself.
- Use reminders or a calendar to build the habit until it becomes routine.

3. Progress at Your Pace

- Beginners should start with modified versions of exercises, such as performing planks on the knees or slowing down mountain climbers.
- Over time, increase intensity by incorporating resistance bands, adding weights, or extending work intervals.

4. Track Your Progress

- Keep a journal or use an app to track your workouts, reps, and how you feel after each session. Seeing your progress will boost motivation.

The Benefits of a Minimalist Approach

- **Accessibility:** Whether you're at home, traveling, or outdoors, you can adapt the workouts to fit your environment.
- **Affordability:** With minimal gear required, the program is cost-effective for any budget.

- **Efficiency:** No need to commute to a gym or wait for equipment—just roll out your mat and get started.

This straightforward, minimalist setup ensures that nothing stands between you and your goals. Now that you're equipped and ready to begin, the next chapters will guide you through the specific workouts designed to burn belly fat and sculpt your core—all in just 15 minutes.

Warm-Up: Essential Routines for Injury Prevention

Warming up is a crucial part of any workout routine, particularly for high-intensity exercises targeting your core. A proper warm-up prepares your body by increasing blood flow, improving flexibility, and reducing the risk of injuries.

Why Warm-Up Matters

- **Increases Body Temperature:** Warmer muscles are more pliable and less prone to strains.
- **Enhances Joint Mobility:** Loosens stiff joints for better range of motion.
- **Activates Core Muscles:** Engages your abdominal muscles, ensuring they're ready for the workout ahead.
- **Improves Mind-Body Connection:** Prepares you mentally for exercise by focusing your attention on movement and form.

5-Minute Warm-Up Routine

Perform each exercise for 30–60 seconds:

1. **Standing Torso Twists:**
   - Stand with feet shoulder-width apart. Twist your upper body side to side, keeping your core engaged.
   - Purpose: Activates obliques and warms up the spine.

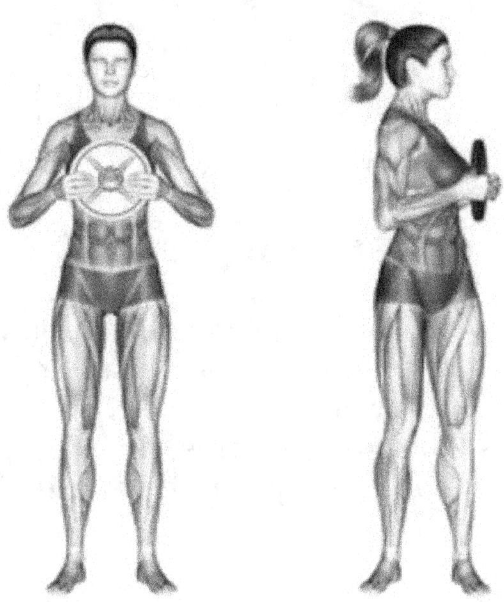

2. **Arm Circles:**
   - Extend your arms out to the sides and make small forward circles, gradually increasing size. Repeat in reverse.

o   Purpose: Loosens shoulders and prepares upper-body stabilizers.

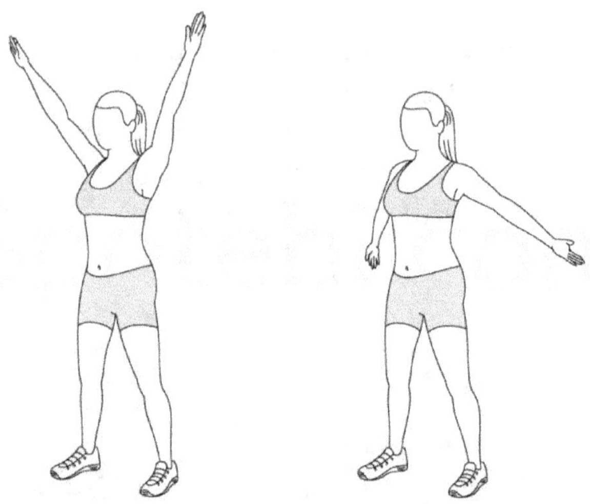

3. **Cat-Cow Stretch:**
   o   Get on all fours, arching your back upward (Cat Pose), then lowering it while lifting your head and tailbone (Cow Pose).
   o   Purpose: Warms up the spine and core while promoting flexibility.

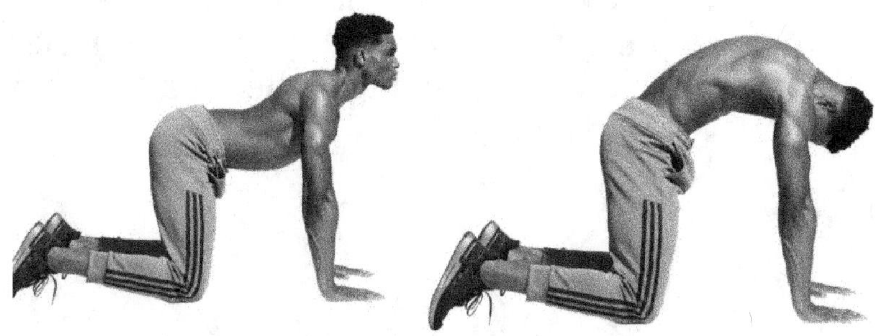

4. **High Knees or Marching:**
    o Lift your knees high toward your chest, alternating legs. Swing your arms for added movement.
    o Purpose: Elevates heart rate and activates lower abdominal muscles.

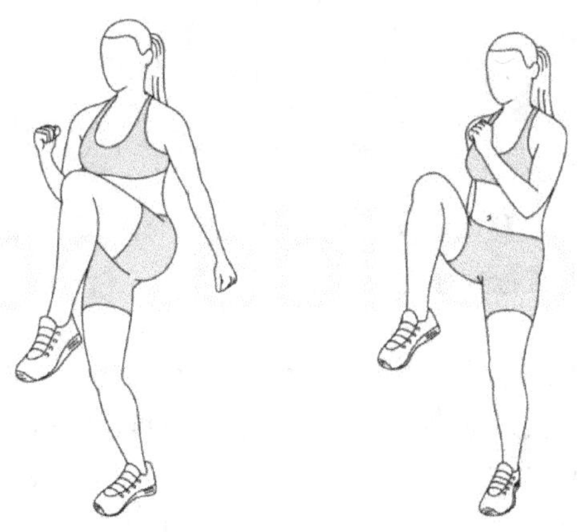

5. **Plank-to-Downward Dog:**

- o Start in a plank position, then push back into Downward Dog. Alternate between the two positions.
  - o Purpose: Activates core muscles while stretching the back and hamstrings.

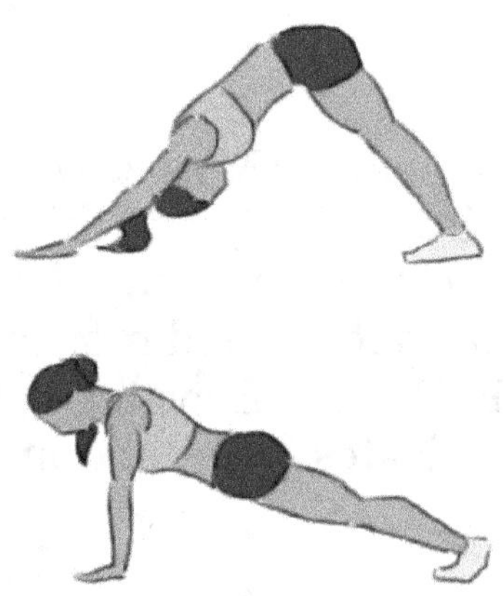

Tracking Progress: Stay Motivated and Monitor Results

To achieve and sustain results with the 15-Minute Flat Belly Fix, it's essential to track your progress. Documenting your journey helps you stay accountable, see tangible improvements, and adjust your program as needed.

Why Tracking Progress is Important

- **Motivation:** Watching your improvements—whether it's stronger abs, better endurance, or a slimmer waist—keeps you inspired.
- **Accountability:** Regularly recording your workouts and measurements ensures you stay consistent.
- **Adjustment:** Tracking helps identify areas for improvement, such as increasing intensity or tweaking your nutrition plan.

Methods for Tracking Progress

1. **Progress Photos**
   - **How to Take Them:**
     - Wear similar clothing each time (e.g., workout gear or swimwear).
     - Take photos from the front, side, and back under the same lighting conditions.
     - Take photos every 2–4 weeks to compare results.
   - **What to Look For:**
     - Changes in muscle definition, waist size, and posture.
2. **Measurements**
   - **Key Areas to Measure:**
     - Waist circumference: Measure around the narrowest part of your torso.
     - Hip circumference: Measure at the widest part of your hips.

- Other areas: Track changes in thighs, arms, or chest if desired.
  - **Frequency:** Measure every 2 weeks for consistent updates.
3. **Fitness Apps and Tools**
   - **Apps to Use:**
     - Fitness trackers (e.g., MyFitnessPal, Fitbit) can log workouts, calories burned, and nutrition.
     - Specialized apps for core workouts offer exercise libraries and progress tracking.
   - **Benefits:** Many apps generate charts or reminders, making it easier to stay on track.
4. **Journal or Workbook**
   - **What to Record:**
     - Date, type of workout, duration, and notes on how you felt.
     - Weekly reflections on progress, challenges, or achievements.
   - **Why It Works:** Writing down your journey creates a personal connection to your goals and highlights your growth over time.

Staying Consistent with Tracking

- **Set a Routine:** Dedicate one day each week to review and log your progress.
- **Celebrate Wins:** Reward yourself for small milestones, like completing a full plank hold or reducing your waist by an inch.
- **Focus on Non-Scale Victories:** Improved posture, better endurance, and increased confidence are just as important as physical changes.

Chapter 5: Beginner Workouts

Starting your fitness journey can feel daunting, but with the 15-Minute Flat Belly Fix, you'll ease into a routine designed to build a solid foundation. This chapter focuses on beginner-friendly workouts tailored to those new to exercise or returning after a long break. These routines emphasize core strength, stability, and proper form to set the stage for long-term success.

Why Start with Beginner Workouts?

1. **Build Core Strength Gradually:**
   - Avoid injury by starting with movements that prepare your muscles, joints, and connective tissues for more challenging exercises.
2. **Master Proper Form:**
   - Learning correct techniques ensures effectiveness and prevents strain, especially in the lower back.
3. **Boost Confidence:**
   - Simple yet effective routines make it easier to stay consistent and motivated.
4. **Promote Long-Term Progress:**
   - A strong foundation allows you to progress to more advanced movements with ease.

Key Principles for Beginners

1. **Focus on Stability Over Speed:**
   - Perform each movement with control, prioritizing proper form over the number of reps.
2. **Engage Your Core:**
   - Always tighten your abdominal muscles during exercises. Think of pulling your belly button toward your spine.
3. **Breathe Effectively:**
   - Exhale during exertion (e.g., lifting or crunching) and inhale during relaxation phases.
4. **Take Breaks When Needed:**
   - Pause briefly if your form starts to waver. Quality over quantity is key.

15-Minute Beginner Core Routine

Perform each exercise for 30 seconds, resting for 10–15 seconds between exercises. Complete 2 rounds for a full 15-minute session.

Warm-Up (2 Minutes)

- **Cat-Cow Stretch (30 seconds):** Loosens the spine and warms up the core.

- **Marching in Place (30 seconds):** Raises your heart rate gently.
- **Torso Twists (30 seconds):** Engages obliques and improves spinal mobility.

Workout (10 Minutes)

1. **Knee Tucks (Modified Plank)**

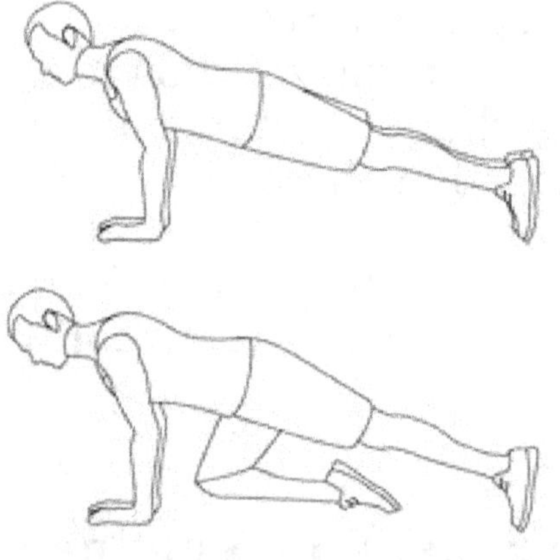

- **How to Do It:**
  - Begin in a tabletop position on all fours.
  - Pull one knee toward your chest, engaging your core, and return to starting position. Alternate legs.
- **Benefits:** Builds core stability and improves coordination.

2. Dead Bug

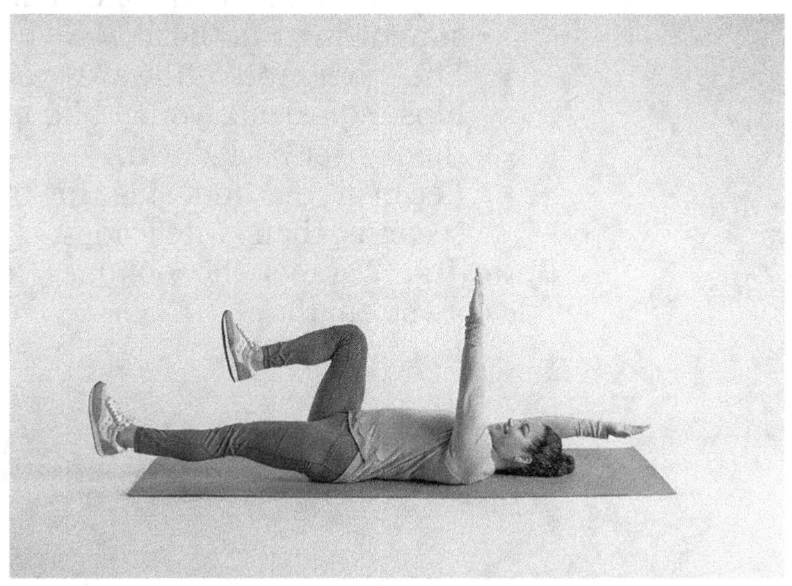

- o **How to Do It:**
  - Lie on your back with arms extended toward the ceiling and knees bent at 90 degrees.
  - Slowly lower your right arm and left leg toward the floor, keeping your core engaged. Return to starting position and switch sides.
- o **Benefits:** Strengthens the deep core muscles without straining the neck or back.

3. Side-Lying Oblique Crunches
- o **How to Do It:**

- Lie on your side with legs slightly bent and one hand supporting your head.
- Lift your torso toward your hips, squeezing your obliques, then lower back down.
- Perform on one side for 30 seconds, then switch sides.
  - **Benefits:** Targets the obliques for side core strength.

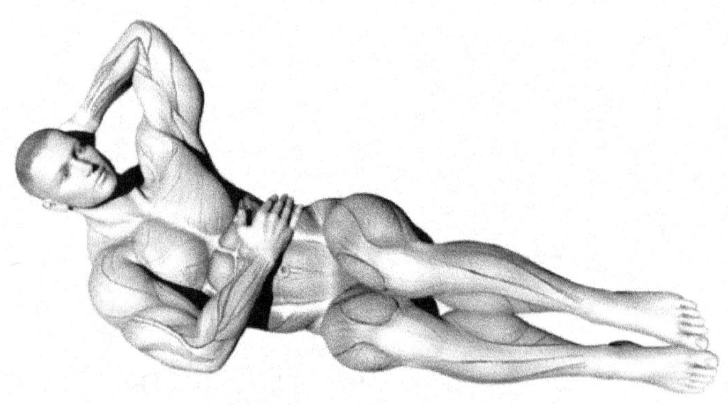

4. Glute Bridge

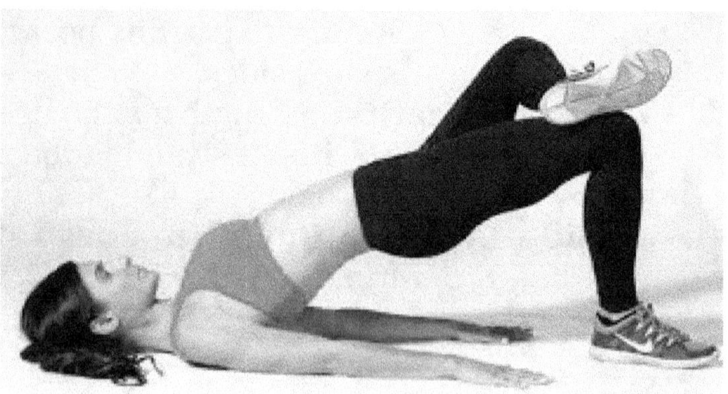

- o **How to Do It:**
  - Lie on your back with knees bent and feet flat on the floor.
  - Lift your hips toward the ceiling, squeezing your glutes and engaging your core. Slowly lower down.
- o **Benefits:** Strengthens the lower back, glutes, and deep abdominal muscles.

5. **Seated Leg Lifts**

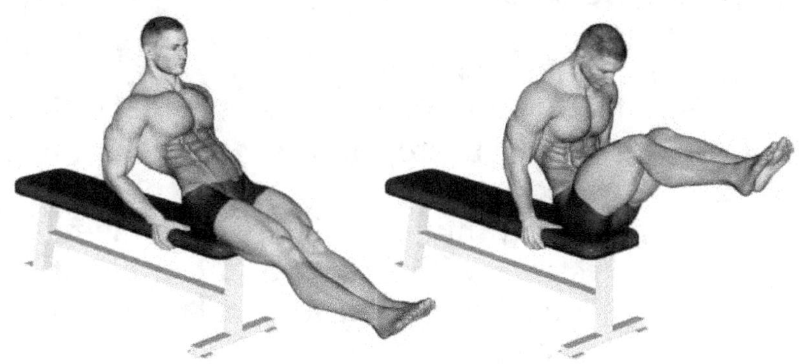

- o **How to Do It:**
  - Sit on the floor with hands resting beside your hips for support.
  - Lift one leg a few inches off the ground, hold for a second, and lower. Alternate legs.
- o **Benefits:** Builds lower abdominal strength gently.

Cool Down (3 Minutes)

1. **Child's Pose (30 seconds):** Stretch out the back and relax your core muscles.
2. **Seated Forward Fold (30 seconds):** Stretch the hamstrings and lower back.
3. **Knees-to-Chest Stretch (30 seconds):** Release tension in the lower back and hips.

Tips for Beginners

1. **Listen to Your Body:**
   - Discomfort is okay, but pain is a signal to stop and reassess your form.
2. **Start Slow:**
   - If 15 minutes feels overwhelming, start with one round (about 8 minutes total) and gradually increase.
3. **Focus on Consistency:**
   - Completing a few effective workouts each week is better than doing too much and burning out.
4. **Track Progress:**
   - Record how you feel after each workout. As you get stronger, you'll notice improved stability and endurance.

Building Toward More Advanced Workouts

After mastering the beginner routine and building a strong foundation, you'll be ready to progress to intermediate and advanced workouts. These will incorporate higher intensity, dynamic movements, and resistance for continued results.

By starting with this beginner plan, you're not only strengthening your core but also setting yourself up for long-term success in your journey to a flatter belly and a stronger body.

Sample Beginner Workout: Core Foundation Routine

This quick, beginner-friendly workout focuses on foundational core exercises to build strength and stability. It's designed to be simple yet effective, allowing you to ease into your fitness journey.

Workout Structure

- Perform each exercise for the prescribed time or repetitions.
- Rest for 30–60 seconds after completing all exercises in the set.
- Repeat the entire circuit 2–3 times, depending on your fitness level.

1. Plank Hold (30 seconds)

- **How to Do It:**
    1. Start in a forearm plank position, with elbows directly under shoulders and legs extended straight behind you.
    2. Engage your core, keeping your body in a straight line from head to heels.
    3. Avoid arching your back or letting your hips drop.
    4. Hold for 30 seconds, breathing steadily.
- **Benefits:**
  Strengthens the entire core, including the rectus abdominis, transverse abdominis, and lower back muscles.

---

2. Dead Bug (10 reps per side)

- **How to Do It:**
    1. Lie on your back with arms extended toward the ceiling and knees bent at 90 degrees.
    2. Slowly lower your right arm and left leg toward the floor, keeping your core engaged and your lower back pressed into the ground.
    3. Return to the starting position and repeat on the other side.
    4. Perform 10 reps per side.

- **Benefits:**
  Targets deep core muscles, improving stability and coordination while reducing strain on the spine.

3. Glute Bridge (10 reps)

- **How to Do It:**
  1. Lie on your back with knees bent and feet flat on the floor, hip-width apart.
  2. Press through your heels to lift your hips toward the ceiling, squeezing your glutes and engaging your core at the top.
  3. Slowly lower back down to the starting position.
  4. Perform 10 repetitions.
- **Benefits:**
  Strengthens the lower back, glutes, and core while improving hip mobility and reducing lower back discomfort.

4. Rest and Repeat

- Rest for 30–60 seconds after completing the set.
- Repeat the circuit 2–3 times, based on your fitness level and comfort.

Tips for the Workout

1. **Modify as Needed:**
    o   For the plank, drop to your knees if maintaining a full plank is too challenging.
    o   For the glute bridge, place a pillow under your lower back for added support if needed.
2. **Focus on Form:**
    o   Quality over quantity! Ensure proper alignment and core engagement for each exercise.
3. **Progress Gradually:**
    o   As you build strength, try extending the plank duration, increasing the number of reps, or reducing rest time between circuits.

Why This Routine Works

- **Time-Efficient:** Takes just 10–15 minutes to complete, perfect for busy schedules.
- **Core-Focused:** Targets multiple core muscles, ensuring balanced strength development.
- **Beginner-Friendly:** Simple, low-impact movements minimize strain while building a strong foundation.

By incorporating this routine into your fitness plan, you'll be taking the first steps toward a flatter belly and stronger core. As you gain confidence and strength, you'll be ready to tackle more advanced workouts in later chapters.

Chapter 6: Intermediate Workouts

Once you've built a solid foundation with beginner exercises, it's time to elevate your routine with more dynamic movements. Intermediate workouts focus on enhancing fat burning, improving endurance, and toning your abdominal muscles. These routines are designed to challenge your core stability while adding intensity to boost calorie burn and sculpt your midsection.

Why Transition to Intermediate Workouts?

1. **Increase Fat Burning:**
   - More dynamic movements raise your heart rate, increasing caloric expenditure during and after the workout (EPOC effect).
2. **Enhance Core Engagement:**
   - Complex exercises activate multiple muscle groups, including the deeper core muscles.
3. **Build Endurance:**
   - Intermediate workouts improve stamina, preparing you for advanced routines.
4. **Tone and Define Muscles:**
   - These movements target not just the abs but also the obliques, hips, and

lower back, leading to a more sculpted core.

Key Principles for Intermediate Workouts

1. **Incorporate Compound Movements:**
   - Engage multiple muscle groups for maximum efficiency.
2. **Maintain Good Form:**
   - Control each movement to avoid injury and ensure proper muscle activation.
3. **Increase Intensity Gradually:**
   - Add reps, sets, or duration over time as your fitness improves.
4. **Focus on Core and Cardiovascular Blend:**
   - Combine static holds, dynamic movements, and cardio bursts for balanced results.

15-Minute Intermediate Core Routine

This workout blends fat-burning cardio with core-strengthening exercises. Perform each exercise for the prescribed reps or time, rest for 30–60 seconds after the set, and repeat the circuit 2–3 times.

1. Bicycle Crunches (20 reps)

- **How to Do It:**
  1. Lie on your back with hands lightly supporting your head and legs lifted off the ground.
  2. Bring your right elbow toward your left knee as you extend your right leg straight.
  3. Switch sides, bringing your left elbow toward your right knee.
  4. Perform 20 reps (10 per side).
- **Benefits:**
  Targets the obliques and rectus abdominis while improving coordination and flexibility.

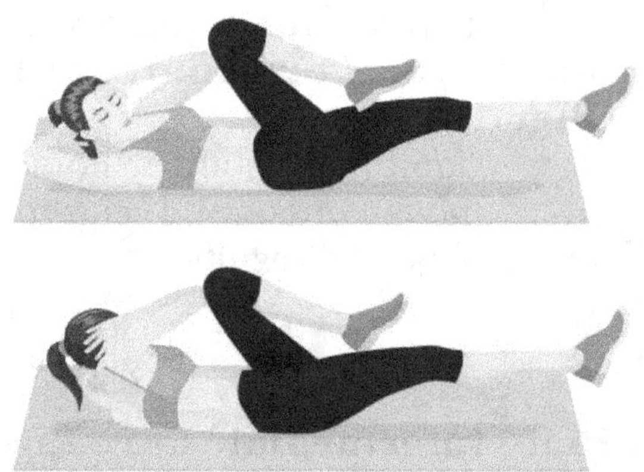

---

2. Side Plank with Hip Dips (10 reps each side)

- **How to Do It:**

1. Begin in a side plank position with your elbow directly under your shoulder, feet stacked, and body in a straight line.
2. Lower your hip toward the floor, then lift it back to the starting position.
3. Perform 10 reps on one side, then switch to the other.

- **Benefits:**
Strengthens the obliques, improves shoulder stability, and challenges balance.

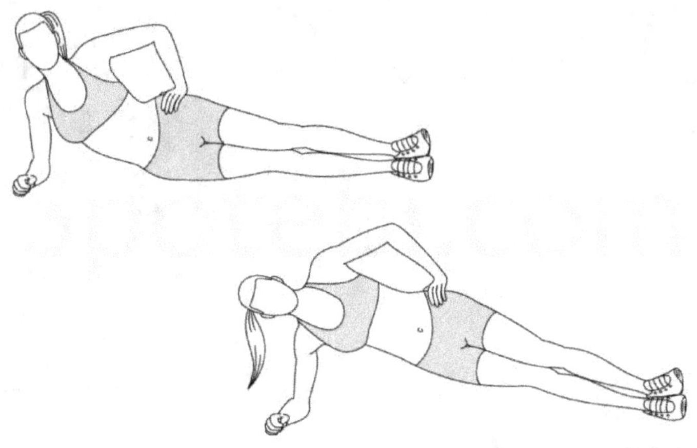

3. Mountain Climbers (30 seconds)

- **How to Do It:**
    1. Start in a high plank position with hands directly under shoulders and body in a straight line.

2. Drive your knees alternately toward your chest as quickly as possible, keeping your core engaged.
3. Perform for 30 seconds.

- **Benefits:**
Combines cardio and core engagement, boosting heart rate and calorie burn.

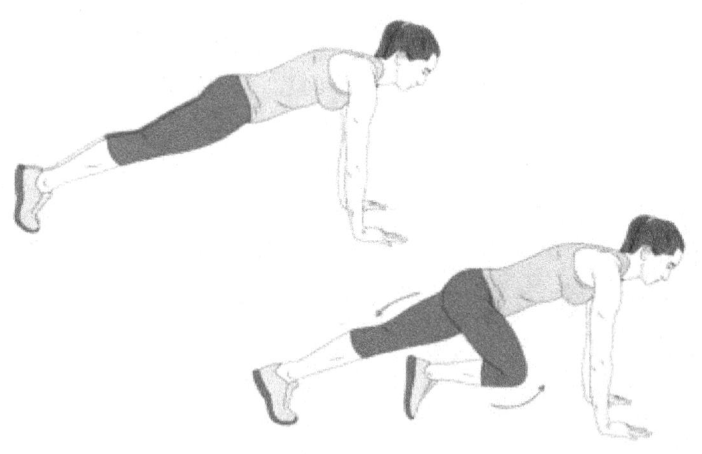

4. Rest and Repeat

- Rest for 30–60 seconds after completing the circuit.
- Repeat the entire set 2–3 times, depending on your fitness level and energy.

Tips for Success

1. **Maintain Proper Alignment:**
   - For bicycle crunches and mountain climbers, avoid arching your lower back to protect your spine.
2. **Control the Tempo:**
   - Perform movements at a steady pace to ensure proper form, even during cardio exercises like mountain climbers.
3. **Challenge Yourself:**
   - If the workout becomes too easy, increase reps, add resistance (e.g., ankle weights), or extend plank durations.
4. **Hydrate and Cool Down:**
   - Drink water before and after the session, and always stretch to relax worked muscles.

Why This Routine Works

- **Fat Burning:** Mountain climbers add a cardiovascular component, boosting your metabolism.
- **Core Sculpting:** Bicycle crunches and side planks tone the abdominal muscles for a more defined look.
- **Intermediate Challenge:** The variety of movements keeps the workout engaging and progressively challenges your core strength.

By completing this intermediate routine consistently, you'll notice improved endurance, better posture, and more visible muscle definition. These gains will prepare you for the advanced workouts in the next phase of your journey.

Chapter 7: Advanced Workouts

Unleashing Your Potential with Advanced Core Workouts

Congratulations on reaching the advanced stage of your core training journey! This chapter focuses on high-intensity routines designed to push your limits, burn maximum fat, and achieve the sculpted core you've been working toward. Advanced workouts demand focus, stamina, and proper form. By integrating complex movements, we'll challenge your strength, endurance, and coordination, ensuring you continue to progress.

High-Intensity Routines: Maximizing Fat Burn and Core Definition

Advanced core workouts combine strength training with explosive, full-body movements to create a powerful fat-burning effect. These routines elevate your heart rate, increase calorie expenditure, and engage multiple muscle groups simultaneously.

Benefits of High-Intensity Advanced Core Routines:

1. **Maximized Calorie Burn:** Incorporating high-intensity exercises like burpees and hanging leg raises activates your

metabolism, promoting fat loss during and after your workout.

2. **Enhanced Muscle Definition:** The intensity and variety of these exercises target deep core muscles, building strength and revealing definition.
3. **Improved Functional Fitness:** Advanced movements improve coordination, balance, and overall athletic performance.
4. **Mental Toughness:** Pushing through high-intensity routines builds mental resilience and confidence in your abilities.

Guidelines for Success in Advanced Workouts

1. **Warm-Up Thoroughly:**
   - Prepare your body with a dynamic warm-up to increase blood flow, loosen muscles, and reduce the risk of injury.
   - Example: 5 minutes of light cardio (jumping jacks, jogging in place) and dynamic stretches like torso twists and hip openers.
2. **Focus on Form:**
   - Maintain proper alignment to avoid injury and maximize the effectiveness of each movement. Quality always trumps quantity.
3. **Listen to Your Body:**

- o Advanced workouts are challenging. Take short breaks or modify exercises if needed but aim to push your limits.
4. **Stay Consistent:**
   - o Advanced routines are demanding, but regular practice ensures continuous improvement and results.

Sample Advanced Workout: The Fat-Burning Core Circuit

This high-intensity circuit is designed to work your entire core while promoting fat loss. Perform each exercise with focus and control. Rest briefly between exercises, then repeat the circuit for maximum impact.

Circuit Overview:

- **Burpees with Push-Up (10 reps)**
- **Russian Twists (20 reps with weight)**
- **Hanging Leg Raises (12 reps)**
- **Rest for 1-2 minutes, then repeat 3-5 rounds**

Detailed Exercise Breakdown:

1. Burpees with Push-Up (10 reps)
This powerhouse exercise combines cardio and

strength, working your core, chest, arms, and legs while spiking your heart rate.

- **Execution:**
    1. Start in a standing position.
    2. Drop into a squat, placing your hands on the floor.
    3. Kick your feet back into a plank position.
    4. Perform a push-up, keeping your core tight and back straight.
    5. Jump your feet back to the squat position.
    6. Explode upward into a jump, reaching your hands overhead.
- **Tips:**

    o Maintain a strong plank during the push-up.
    o Land softly when jumping to reduce impact.

Modification:
    o Skip the jump for a lower-impact version.

---

2. Russian Twists (20 reps with weight)
Targeting the obliques, Russian twists sculpt your waistline while improving rotational strength.

- **Execution:**

1. Sit on the floor with knees bent and feet lifted off the ground (or keep them grounded for stability).
2. Hold a weight (e.g., a dumbbell or medicine ball) with both hands.
3. Lean back slightly to engage your core.
4. Twist your torso to the right, bringing the weight toward the floor.
5. Return to the center, then twist to the left.

- **Tips:**

  - Keep your movements controlled; avoid letting momentum take over.
  - Engage your core throughout to protect your lower back.

Modification:
  - Perform without weight to reduce intensity.

---

3. Hanging Leg Raises (12 reps)
This challenging move strengthens the lower abs while engaging the entire core.

- **Execution:**
  1. Hang from a pull-up bar with an overhand grip, arms fully extended.
  2. Keep your legs straight and together.
  3. Engage your core to lift your legs until they're parallel to the ground.

4. Slowly lower your legs back to the starting position.

- **Tips:**

  - Avoid swinging; use controlled movements.
  - Engage your shoulder blades to stabilize your upper body.

  Modification:
  - Perform knee raises instead of straight-leg raises.

Rest and Repeat

After completing the circuit, take a 1-2 minute rest to allow your heart rate to recover. Repeat the circuit 3-5 times based on your fitness level and endurance. Gradually aim to reduce rest times as you build stamina.

Post-Workout Stretching and Recovery

Advanced workouts place a significant demand on your muscles. Conclude with a stretching routine focused on the core and hip flexors to prevent stiffness and promote recovery.

- **Examples:**
  - **Cobra Stretch:** To lengthen the abdominal muscles.

- o **Cat-Cow Pose:** To release tension in the lower back.
- o **Child's Pose:** To stretch and relax the entire core.

By incorporating high-intensity circuits like this one into your routine, you'll continue to challenge yourself, burn fat, and achieve remarkable core definition. Push hard, stay consistent, and celebrate the strength you're building with every workout!

Chapter 8: The Weekly Workout Schedule

A strong, defined core doesn't come from sporadic effort; it's built through a well-structured, balanced, and consistent workout schedule. This chapter provides you with a framework for organizing your weekly workouts to optimize results, blending core-specific exercises, full-body strength training, and cardio. Recovery strategies are also covered to ensure sustainable progress and minimize injury risk.

How to Structure Workouts for Optimal Results

A balanced workout schedule targets all muscle groups, prioritizes core engagement, and incorporates variety to prevent plateaus. Here's how to effectively structure your week:

Key Principles of Weekly Workout Planning:

1. **Focus on Variety:** Alternate between core-focused days, full-body strength training, and cardio to maximize results.
2. **Progressive Overload:** Gradually increase intensity by adding reps, sets, or resistance to challenge your muscles.
3. **Include Recovery:** Incorporate active recovery days to allow muscles to repair and grow.

4. **Schedule Consistency:** Aim for 4-6 workout days per week, tailored to your fitness level and goals.

Sample Weekly Workout Schedule

Day 1: Core and Cardio Blast

- Warm-Up: 5 minutes (dynamic stretches, light cardio)
- Circuit:
    - Burpees with Push-Up (10 reps)
    - Russian Twists (20 reps with weight)
    - High Knees (30 seconds)
    - Plank Hold (60 seconds)
- Cool-Down: 5 minutes (stretching)

Day 2: Full-Body Strength Training

- Warm-Up: 5 minutes (jump rope, arm circles)
- Exercises:
    - Deadlifts (3 sets of 12 reps)
    - Push-Ups (3 sets of 15 reps)
    - Goblet Squats (3 sets of 10 reps)
    - Dumbbell Rows (3 sets of 12 reps per arm)
- Cool-Down: 5 minutes (focus on hamstring and shoulder stretches)

Day 3: Active Recovery and Mobility

- Yoga or Pilates session focusing on core recovery and flexibility.
- Stretches: Cobra, Seated Twist, and Child's Pose.

Day 4: High-Intensity Core Circuit

- Warm-Up: 5 minutes (jumping jacks, arm swings)
- Circuit:
  - Plank Jacks (12 reps)
  - Hanging Leg Raises (12 reps)
  - Mountain Climbers (30 seconds)
  - Bicycle Crunches (15 reps per side)
- Cool-Down: 5 minutes (core and lower back stretches)

Day 5: Cardio and Core Combo

- Warm-Up: 5 minutes (light jogging or stationary bike)
- Routine:
  - 20 minutes of moderate cardio (running, cycling, or swimming)
  - Core Finisher:
    - Side Planks (30 seconds per side)
    - Flutter Kicks (20 reps)
- Cool-Down: 5 minutes (stretching)

Day 6: Full-Body Functional Training

- Warm-Up: 5 minutes (jump rope, dynamic lunges)

- Exercises:
  - Kettlebell Swings (3 sets of 15 reps)
  - Dumbbell Shoulder Press (3 sets of 12 reps)
  - Bulgarian Split Squats (3 sets of 10 reps per leg)
  - Renegade Rows (3 sets of 12 reps)
- Cool-Down: 5 minutes (focus on hips, chest, and hamstrings)

Day 7: Rest or Light Activity

- Take a full rest day or engage in a light activity like walking or stretching to keep the body moving while allowing recovery.

Combining Ab Workouts with Full-Body Strength and Cardio

Why the Combination Works:

1. **Core Integration:** Many full-body exercises (like deadlifts and squats) naturally engage the core. Adding targeted ab workouts ensures comprehensive muscle activation.
2. **Fat Loss Synergy:** Cardio aids in calorie burning, while strength training boosts metabolism, complementing core-focused routines for visible results.

3. **Balanced Development:** A mix of these elements prevents overtraining specific areas, reducing injury risk.

Practical Tips:

- Include 10-15 minutes of focused ab work at the end of strength training or cardio sessions.
- Prioritize exercises that complement each other; for example, pairing squats with planks or push-ups with Russian twists.

Rest and Recovery Strategies

Recovery is a critical part of any fitness program, especially for advanced routines that challenge your muscles and endurance. Proper recovery allows your core and entire body to rebuild stronger and more resilient.

Key Recovery Practices:

1. **Active Recovery:** Engage in low-intensity activities like yoga, walking, or stretching to maintain blood flow and muscle mobility.
2. **Hydration and Nutrition:** Replenish lost fluids and fuel muscle repair with nutrient-rich foods. Include protein for muscle repair and carbohydrates for energy.

3. **Stretching:** Incorporate core-specific stretches like the Cobra, Cat-Cow, and Seated Forward Fold post-workout.
4. **Sleep:** Ensure 7-9 hours of quality sleep to support overall recovery and performance.

By following this structured schedule and adhering to recovery strategies, you'll optimize your results, maintain consistency, and set yourself up for long-term success. With a balanced approach, every week becomes a step closer to achieving a leaner, stronger core.

Part 3: Nutrition for a Flat Belly

A toned midsection is not just about exercise—it's heavily influenced by what you eat. Nutrition plays a critical role in losing belly fat, promoting muscle definition, and improving overall health. This part of the book explores how diet supports a flat belly by focusing on calorie balance, fat-burning foods, and avoiding harmful dietary choices.

Chapter 9: The Role of Nutrition in Belly Fat Loss

In this chapter, we delve into the fundamentals of nutrition for shedding stubborn belly fat. By understanding the principles of calorie management, incorporating foods that boost metabolism, and avoiding detrimental dietary pitfalls, you can create a sustainable path to achieving your fitness goals.

Calories In vs. Calories Out

The cornerstone of fat loss is achieving a calorie deficit—burning more calories than you consume. Here's how it works:

- **Energy Balance:**

- o When you consume more calories than you burn, excess energy is stored as fat, often around the belly.
    - o Consuming fewer calories than your body needs forces it to tap into fat reserves for energy.
- **Key Steps for Calorie Management:**
    - o **Determine Your Basal Metabolic Rate (BMR):** This is the number of calories your body needs to maintain basic functions.
    - o **Track Your Intake:** Use apps or food journals to monitor daily caloric consumption.
    - o **Incorporate Exercise:** Combining a healthy diet with physical activity accelerates calorie burning.

Example:

- If your BMR is 1,800 calories and you add moderate exercise that burns 300 calories, you should aim for a daily intake of about 1,800-2,000 calories to create a deficit without depriving your body.

Foods That Promote Fat Burning

Certain foods naturally enhance fat burning by boosting metabolism, curbing appetite, or reducing inflammation. Incorporating these into your diet can accelerate belly fat loss.

1. **Protein:**
   - o **Why It Works:** Protein has a high thermic effect, meaning your body burns more calories digesting it. It also promotes satiety and muscle preservation during weight loss.
   - o **Sources:** Lean meats, eggs, tofu, Greek yogurt, legumes, and fish like salmon.
2. **Healthy Fats:**
   - o **Why It Works:** Unsaturated fats help regulate hormones that control appetite and fat storage.
   - o **Sources:** Avocado, nuts, seeds, olive oil, and fatty fish.
3. **Fiber:**
   - o **Why It Works:** High-fiber foods slow digestion, keeping you full longer and stabilizing blood sugar levels.
   - o **Sources:** Oats, quinoa, fruits like berries, vegetables, and legumes.
4. **Thermogenic Foods:**
   - o **Why It Works:** Spices like cayenne pepper and ginger slightly raise body temperature, increasing calorie burn.
   - o **Sources:** Green tea, black coffee (in moderation), cinnamon, and turmeric.

Foods to Avoid

To minimize belly fat, steer clear of foods that lead to weight gain, inflammation, and bloating.

1. **Refined Sugars:**
   - Found in soda, candy, and baked goods, these spike blood sugar levels, leading to increased fat storage.
2. **Trans Fats:**
   - Found in some margarine, fried foods, and packaged snacks, trans fats promote inflammation and abdominal fat storage.
3. **Processed Snacks:**
   - Chips, crackers, and pre-packaged sweets often contain empty calories, unhealthy fats, and excess sodium that contribute to bloating and fat gain.
4. **Excessive Alcohol:**
   - "Empty" calories from alcohol can quickly add up, and excessive drinking disrupts fat metabolism, particularly in the abdominal area.

Practical Tips for Belly Fat Loss

1. **Plan Your Meals:** Avoid last-minute unhealthy choices by preparing balanced meals ahead of time.
2. **Stay Hydrated:** Drinking water throughout the day helps control appetite and supports digestion.

3. **Practice Portion Control:** Even healthy foods can lead to weight gain if consumed in excessive amounts. Use smaller plates or portion out snacks to avoid overeating.
4. **Mind Your Cooking Methods:** Opt for grilling, steaming, or baking over frying to reduce unnecessary calories and fats.

Dinner: Light Yet Satisfying Dishes

Dinner is the perfect time to focus on nutrient-dense meals that provide protein, healthy fats, and fiber while keeping calories in check. Here are some belly-fat-friendly dinner ideas:

1. Baked Salmon with Steamed Veggies

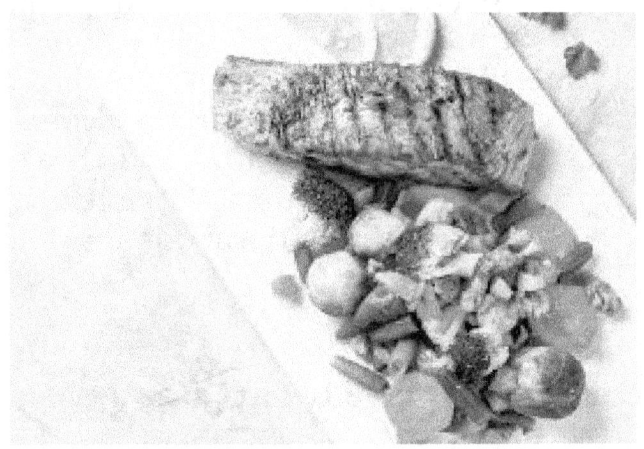

- **Why It Works:** Salmon is rich in omega-3 fatty acids, which help reduce inflammation and promote fat metabolism, while steamed vegetables add fiber and essential nutrients.
- **Recipe Idea:**

- o 4 oz salmon filet, seasoned with garlic, lemon juice, and dill
- o Steamed broccoli, carrots, and asparagus
- o A drizzle of olive oil or a squeeze of fresh lemon juice over the veggies
- o Serve with a side of quinoa or cauliflower rice for added texture.

2. Grilled Chicken with Zucchini Noodles

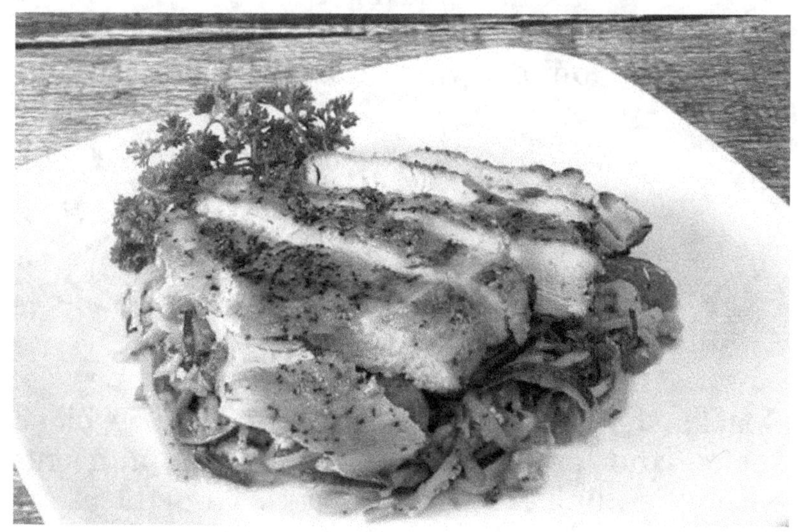

- **Why It Works:** High-protein chicken paired with low-carb zucchini noodles makes for a light yet filling dish.
- **Recipe Idea:**
  - o 4 oz grilled chicken breast, seasoned with paprika and herbs
  - o 2 cups zucchini spirals sautéed in olive oil with minced garlic

o Top with a sprinkle of Parmesan cheese and fresh basil

3. Lentil and Vegetable Stir-Fry

- **Why It Works:** Lentils are a plant-based protein powerhouse, and the fiber in the stir-fried vegetables helps improve digestion and reduce bloating.
- **Recipe Idea:**
    o ½ cup cooked lentils
    o Sautéed bell peppers, snap peas, onions, and mushrooms in sesame oil
    o Add a splash of soy sauce or coconut aminos for flavor

Snacks: Belly-Fat-Friendly Ideas

Snacks should help curb hunger, stabilize blood sugar, and provide a quick dose of nutrients without adding excessive calories. These ideas are simple, portable, and effective for supporting your flat-belly goals.

1. Almonds

- **Why It Works:** Almonds are packed with healthy fats, protein, and fiber to keep you feeling full and satisfied.
- **Serving Size:** 1 small handful (about 12-15 almonds)

- **Tip:** Opt for unsalted or lightly salted almonds to avoid unnecessary sodium intake.

2. Boiled Eggs

- **Why It Works:** Eggs are rich in high-quality protein and essential nutrients like choline, which supports metabolism.
- **Serving Size:** 1-2 boiled eggs
- **Tip:** Sprinkle with a pinch of sea salt or paprika for added flavor.

3. Greek Yogurt with a Drizzle of Honey

- **Why It Works:** Greek yogurt provides probiotics for gut health, while a touch of honey satisfies sweet cravings without processed sugars.
- **Serving Size:** ½ cup plain Greek yogurt with ½ teaspoon honey
- **Tip:** Add a few sliced almonds or a sprinkle of cinnamon for extra flavor and texture.

4. Veggie Sticks with Hummus

- **Why It Works:** Fresh vegetables like carrots, celery, and cucumber are hydrating and low in calories, while hummus adds a boost of healthy fats and plant-based protein.
- **Serving Size:** 1 cup mixed veggie sticks with 2 tablespoons hummus

- **Tip:** Choose a hummus flavor like roasted garlic or red pepper for variety.

5. Dark Chocolate Squares

- **Why It Works:** A small portion of dark chocolate (70% cacao or higher) satisfies chocolate cravings while providing antioxidants.
- **Serving Size:** 1-2 small squares (about 1 oz)
- **Tip:** Pair with a handful of berries for a sweet and nutrient-rich treat.

Tips for Meal Timing and Portion Control

1. **Dinner Timing:** Aim to eat dinner at least 2-3 hours before bedtime to allow your body to digest properly and avoid late-night bloating.
2. **Snack Strategy:** Incorporate snacks mid-morning or mid-afternoon to maintain steady energy levels and prevent overeating at main meals.
3. **Portion Awareness:** Use smaller plates for dinner and pre-portion snacks to avoid mindless eating.

Nutritional Highlights

- **Protein:** Central to muscle recovery and fat metabolism.
- **Healthy Fats:** Supports hormone regulation and long-lasting satiety.
- **Fiber:** Promotes digestion and reduces bloating for a leaner appearance.

Chapter 10: Hydration and Detox Tips

Hydration plays a pivotal role in achieving and maintaining a flat belly. It aids in digestion, boosts metabolism, and flushes out toxins, helping to reduce bloating and enhance overall well-being. This chapter explores the science behind hydration and introduces flat-belly-friendly drinks that can support your goals.

The Importance of Water for Digestion and Fat Metabolism

1. Water and Digestion

- **Hydration Supports Digestive Function:** Water helps break down food, allowing your body to absorb nutrients efficiently. Staying hydrated prevents constipation, which can cause bloating and discomfort.
- **Flushes Out Toxins:** Adequate water intake helps the kidneys and liver remove waste products, promoting a cleaner internal environment.

2. Water and Fat Metabolism

- **Lipolysis:** This is the process by which the body breaks down fat. Water is essential for lipolysis, as it helps the body utilize stored fat for energy.

- **Thermogenic Effect:** Drinking water can slightly increase metabolism through thermogenesis, where the body uses energy to warm the water to body temperature.

3. Combating Bloating

- **Sodium Balance:** Drinking water can reduce bloating caused by high sodium intake, as it helps flush excess salt from the body.
- **Maintaining Gut Health:** Proper hydration supports the function of beneficial gut bacteria, which aids in digestion and reduces bloating.

Flat Belly Drinks

Certain drinks not only hydrate but also provide additional benefits like reducing inflammation, boosting metabolism, and calming the digestive system. Here are some excellent choices:

1. Green Tea

- **Why It Works:** Green tea is rich in catechins, antioxidants that promote fat burning and reduce belly fat. It also contains a mild amount of caffeine, which boosts metabolism.
- **How to Use:** Drink 2-3 cups of unsweetened green tea daily, preferably in

the morning or early afternoon for an energy boost.

2. Lemon Water

- **Why It Works:** Lemon water is a natural diuretic and detoxifier. The vitamin C in lemons supports digestion and helps in collagen synthesis for skin health.
- **How to Use:** Squeeze half a lemon into a glass of warm water and drink it first thing in the morning to kickstart digestion.

3. Ginger-Infused Drinks

- **Why It Works:** Ginger has anti-inflammatory properties and aids digestion by speeding up gastric emptying. It can also reduce nausea and bloating.
- **How to Use:** Add a few slices of fresh ginger to hot water or tea. Let it steep for 10 minutes before drinking.

4. Cucumber Mint Water

- **Why It Works:** Cucumber is hydrating and rich in antioxidants, while mint soothes the digestive system. Together, they create a refreshing detox drink.
- **How to Use:** Add slices of cucumber and a handful of fresh mint leaves to a pitcher of water. Let it sit in the refrigerator for 2-3 hours before drinking.

5. Apple Cider Vinegar (ACV) Tonic

- **Why It Works:** ACV may help control blood sugar levels and improve digestion. Its acetic acid content has been linked to fat reduction.
- **How to Use:** Mix 1 tablespoon of ACV in a glass of water. Drink it before meals, but limit it to once a day to avoid potential tooth enamel damage.

6. Herbal Teas

- **Why It Works:** Chamomile, peppermint, and dandelion teas soothe the digestive system and reduce bloating.
- **How to Use:** Enjoy 1-2 cups of herbal tea in the evening to promote relaxation and support digestion.

Tips for Staying Hydrated and Detoxifying

1. **Daily Water Goals:** Aim for at least 8-10 glasses (2-2.5 liters) of water daily, adjusting based on activity levels and climate.
2. **Drink Timing:** Start your day with a glass of water and continue to sip throughout the day to maintain hydration. Avoid overdrinking close to bedtime to prevent interrupted sleep.

3. **Add Natural Flavorings:** If plain water feels monotonous, add slices of citrus fruits, berries, or herbs to enhance flavor without added sugars.
4. **Limit Sugary Beverages:** Avoid sodas and fruit juices with added sugar, as they can contribute to weight gain and bloating.

Hydration and Detox Myths: Debunked

- **Myth:** "Detox drinks alone will help you lose belly fat."
  - **Truth:** While certain drinks support digestion and metabolism, they must be combined with a balanced diet and regular exercise for lasting results.
- **Myth:** "More water is always better."
  - **Truth:** Excessive water intake can lead to water intoxication. Drink according to your body's needs.

Hydration is a cornerstone of achieving a flat belly. By incorporating water-rich foods and detoxifying drinks into your daily routine, you can enhance digestion, reduce bloating, and optimize fat metabolism. In the next chapter, we'll combine this knowledge with smart eating strategies to create a flat belly meal plan that fits your lifestyle.

Part 4: Motivation and Lifestyle Habits

Chapter 11: Staying Motivated

Motivation is the driving force behind any fitness or wellness journey, and maintaining it is key to long-term success. This chapter focuses on practical strategies to set achievable goals, recognize progress, and navigate through challenges, helping you stay committed to your flat-belly journey.

Setting Realistic Goals and Tracking Progress

1. Setting SMART Goals

- **Specific:** Define your goals clearly. Instead of "I want a flat belly," try "I want to lose 2 inches from my waistline in 8 weeks."
- **Measurable:** Include metrics such as inches lost, improved endurance, or consistency in workouts.
- **Achievable:** Set goals that challenge you but are realistic given your lifestyle.
- **Relevant:** Ensure your goals align with your broader wellness aspirations, like improved health or increased energy.
- **Time-Bound:** Set a timeframe to keep yourself accountable, e.g., "I will achieve my goal by the end of 12 weeks."

2. Tracking Progress

- **Progress Journals:** Record daily or weekly updates on your workouts, meals, and how you feel physically and mentally.
- **Photos and Measurements:** Take photos and measure your waistline, hips, and weight monthly to track physical changes beyond the scale.
- **Performance Metrics:** Track improvements in endurance, strength, and flexibility through specific exercises like planks or core stretches.
- **Fitness Apps:** Use apps to log workouts, steps, and calorie intake to stay consistent.

Celebrating Small Wins

1. Acknowledge Every Milestone

- Losing an inch, sticking to your meal plan, or completing a challenging workout are victories worth celebrating.
- Celebrate non-scale achievements, such as feeling more energetic, improving your posture, or reducing bloating.

2. Reward Yourself

- Choose rewards that align with your goals, such as buying new workout gear, booking

a massage, or enjoying a guilt-free healthy treat.
- Avoid food-related rewards that contradict your progress, like indulging in sugary snacks.

3. Create a Visual Reminder

- Maintain a visible "victory board" showcasing your milestones to motivate you during challenging days.

Overcoming Plateaus and Setbacks

1. Understanding Plateaus

- **Why They Happen:** Plateaus occur when the body adapts to your routine, leading to slower progress. This is normal in any fitness journey.
- **What to Do:** Introduce new exercises, increase workout intensity, or adjust your nutrition to break through plateaus.

2. Managing Setbacks

- **Recognize They're Normal:** Life events, stress, or illness can disrupt your routine. Understand that setbacks are part of the journey.
- **Refocus Your Mindset:** Shift from an "all-or-nothing" attitude to "progress, not

perfection." Resume your routine as soon as possible.

- **Learn from Challenges:** Identify triggers or habits that led to the setback and plan to address them in the future.

3. Stay Connected for Support

- **Find Accountability Partners:** Partner with a friend, trainer, or online community to stay motivated.
- **Join Fitness Groups:** Engaging with others who share your goals fosters encouragement and shared tips.

Practical Strategies for Staying Motivated

1. Variety in Workouts

- Avoid monotony by trying new activities such as yoga, Pilates, or swimming alongside your core routine.
- Challenge yourself with advanced versions of exercises as you gain strength.

2. Mindset Matters

- Focus on how far you've come rather than how far you still need to go.
- Use positive affirmations to keep your mind engaged and motivated.

3. Create a Routine You Love

- Choose workouts and meals that you genuinely enjoy to ensure long-term adherence.
- Incorporate music, podcasts, or scenic outdoor activities to make your sessions enjoyable.

Motivation isn't a constant; it's a habit you cultivate through small wins, realistic goals, and a positive mindset. By learning to celebrate progress, embrace challenges, and stay flexible, you can keep the momentum alive and continue advancing toward your flat-belly goals.

In the next chapter, we'll explore lifestyle habits that complement your fitness and nutrition efforts, creating a sustainable approach to a healthier, happier you.

Chapter 12: Stress Management for Belly Fat Loss

Stress is one of the most significant yet often overlooked factors in the accumulation of belly fat. This chapter explores the science behind the stress-belly fat connection and provides practical techniques such as yoga, mindfulness, and breathing exercises to help you manage stress and support fat loss.

The Link Between Stress and Belly Fat: Understanding the Cortisol Connection

1. The Role of Cortisol

- **What Is Cortisol?**
  Cortisol is a hormone released by the adrenal glands in response to stress. While it helps the body handle short-term stress, chronic stress causes prolonged cortisol release, which can lead to fat storage.
- **Why Belly Fat?**
  High cortisol levels encourage the body to store fat in the abdominal area, where fat cells have more cortisol receptors. This is part of the "fight or flight" response designed to protect vital organs during stress.

2. Stress Eating

- **Cravings for Comfort Foods:** Chronic stress often triggers cravings for high-calorie, sugary, and fatty foods, which exacerbate belly fat gain.
- **Emotional Eating Patterns:** Stress can disrupt hunger hormones like ghrelin and leptin, leading to overeating and difficulty recognizing fullness.

3. The Stress Cycle

- **Sleep Disruption:** Stress can impair sleep, further elevating cortisol levels and promoting fat storage.
- **Vicious Cycle:** Stress leads to fat gain, which can cause more stress and perpetuate the cycle.

Yoga, Mindfulness, and Breathing Exercises to Manage Stress

1. Yoga for Stress Relief

Yoga combines physical movement with mindful breathing, making it an excellent practice for reducing cortisol levels and promoting relaxation.

Key Stress-Relief Poses:

- **Child's Pose (Balasana):** Promotes relaxation by gently stretching the lower back and calming the nervous system.

- **Legs-Up-the-Wall Pose (Viparita Karani):** Encourages circulation and reduces cortisol levels.
- **Cat-Cow Stretch (Marjaryasana-Bitilasana):** Relieves tension in the spine and improves focus.

Yoga Tips for Stress Management:

- Practice 15–20 minutes of yoga daily or incorporate short routines during breaks to ease stress.
- Focus on poses that emphasize deep stretching and diaphragmatic breathing.

---

2. Mindfulness Techniques

Mindfulness helps you become more aware of your thoughts and feelings, breaking the cycle of stress-induced overeating or negative self-talk.

How to Practice Mindfulness:

- **Mindful Eating:** Slow down during meals, chew thoroughly, and focus on the flavors and textures of food.
- **Body Scans:** Spend 5–10 minutes daily scanning your body for areas of tension, and consciously relax them.
- **Meditation Apps:** Use guided meditation apps like Calm or Headspace to build mindfulness habits.

3. Breathing Exercises to Reduce Stress

Controlled breathing signals the brain to activate the parasympathetic nervous system, countering the stress response and lowering cortisol levels.

Effective Breathing Techniques:

- **Diaphragmatic Breathing (Belly Breathing):**
    - Sit or lie down in a comfortable position.
    - Place one hand on your belly and one on your chest.
    - Breathe deeply through your nose, ensuring your belly rises more than your chest.
    - Exhale slowly through your mouth.
    - Practice for 5–10 minutes daily.
- **Box Breathing:**
    - Inhale for 4 seconds, hold for 4 seconds, exhale for 4 seconds, and hold again for 4 seconds.
    - Repeat for 3–5 minutes to calm your mind and body.
- **Alternate Nostril Breathing (Nadi Shodhana):**
    - Close your right nostril with your thumb, inhale through the left nostril, then close the left nostril and exhale through the right nostril.

o   Continue alternating for 5 minutes to balance energy and reduce stress.

Integrating Stress Management Into Your Routine

- **Morning Routine:** Start your day with 5 minutes of yoga or breathing exercises to set a calming tone.
- **Midday Check-Ins:** Take breaks during work for quick mindfulness or breathing sessions to reset your focus.
- **Evening Wind-Down:** End the day with restorative yoga poses or a short meditation to promote restful sleep.

Conclusion

Stress management isn't just about feeling calmer—it's a vital component of reducing belly fat and improving overall health. By lowering cortisol levels and breaking the cycle of stress eating, practices like yoga, mindfulness, and controlled breathing pave the way for a leaner, healthier you.

In the next chapter, we'll explore how sleep and lifestyle adjustments further enhance your flat-belly journey, building on the foundation of stress reduction.

Chapter 13: Better Sleep for a Flat Belly

A good night's sleep is not just a luxury—it's a crucial factor in your journey to achieving a flat belly. Sleep directly impacts your metabolism, hunger hormones, and fat storage. This chapter explores the science of how sleep influences belly fat and provides actionable tips to improve sleep quality and duration.

How Poor Sleep Affects Metabolism and Fat Storage

1. The Sleep-Metabolism Connection

- **Slower Metabolism:** Inadequate sleep reduces your basal metabolic rate (BMR), making it harder to burn calories even at rest.
- **Insulin Sensitivity:** Poor sleep decreases your body's ability to process glucose, increasing the risk of fat storage, especially in the abdominal area.

2. Hormonal Imbalance

- **Leptin and Ghrelin:** Sleep deprivation lowers leptin (the hormone that signals fullness) and increases ghrelin (the hunger hormone), leading to overeating.

- **Cortisol Levels:** Chronic sleep deficits elevate cortisol, encouraging fat storage in the belly region.

3. Cravings and Overeating

- Lack of sleep triggers cravings for high-calorie, sugary foods, often leading to mindless snacking and overeating.
- Poor sleep also impairs decision-making, making it harder to stick to healthy food choices.

Sleep Hygiene Tips to Improve Quality and Duration

1. Establish a Consistent Sleep Schedule

- **Wake-Up and Bedtime Routine:** Go to bed and wake up at the same time daily, even on weekends. This helps regulate your body's internal clock (circadian rhythm).
- **Avoid Late-Night Disruptions:** Limit late-night screen time and heavy meals, which can delay sleep onset.

---

2. Optimize Your Sleep Environment

- **Darkness and Silence:** Keep your bedroom dark and quiet. Use blackout

curtains, earplugs, or white noise machines if needed.
- **Comfortable Bedding:** Invest in a supportive mattress and comfortable pillows to promote restful sleep.
- **Temperature Control:** Keep the room cool, around 60–67°F (15–19°C), which is ideal for quality sleep.

3. Create a Relaxing Bedtime Routine

- **Wind Down:** Spend 30–60 minutes before bed engaging in relaxing activities like reading, journaling, or gentle yoga.
- **Limit Stimulants:** Avoid caffeine and nicotine 4–6 hours before bedtime, as they can interfere with sleep.
- **Herbal Teas and Essential Oils:** Chamomile tea or lavender essential oil can help signal to your body that it's time to relax.

4. Manage Screen Time

- **The Blue Light Effect:** Blue light from phones, tablets, and computers suppresses melatonin production, the hormone that regulates sleep.

- **Tech-Free Zone:** Avoid screens at least 1 hour before bed or use blue light-blocking glasses if necessary.

5. Incorporate Sleep-Friendly Foods

- **Foods to Include:** Foods high in tryptophan (e.g., turkey, almonds), magnesium (e.g., spinach, bananas), or melatonin (e.g., tart cherries, oats) can promote better sleep.
- **Foods to Avoid:** Limit spicy or acidic foods, alcohol, and heavy meals in the evening to prevent digestive discomfort that disrupts sleep.

6. Stress and Sleep

- Stress and anxiety are common culprits of poor sleep. Techniques such as mindfulness meditation, deep breathing, or progressive muscle relaxation can help calm your mind before bed.

How Better Sleep Supports Belly Fat Loss

- **Improved Metabolism:** Quality sleep enhances your body's ability to burn calories and use energy efficiently.
- **Hormonal Balance:** Restful sleep regulates hunger and stress hormones, reducing cravings and overeating.
- **Workout Recovery:** Sleep promotes muscle recovery and energy replenishment, enabling you to perform better in workouts.

Simple Sleep Improvement Checklist

1. Stick to a consistent bedtime and wake-up schedule.
2. Keep your bedroom cool, dark, and quiet.
3. Limit screen time before bed and create a relaxing pre-sleep routine.
4. Include calming foods and avoid stimulants in the evening.
5. Use mindfulness or relaxation techniques to manage stress.

Quality sleep is a cornerstone of both physical and mental health, playing a pivotal role in achieving a leaner, healthier body. By prioritizing sleep hygiene, you'll not only boost your metabolism and reduce belly fat but also improve your overall well-being.

In the next chapter, we'll explore how consistent habits and long-term strategies can help you sustain your progress and maintain a flat belly for life.

Part 5: Long-Term Results and Maintenance

Chapter 14: Transitioning to a Sustainable Routine

Achieving a flat belly is an empowering journey, but maintaining that result is where the true challenge lies. In this chapter, we'll explore how to make your progress last by transitioning into a sustainable routine that keeps you motivated, engaged, and physically fit long after your initial results. Whether you've been following the 15-minute plan or have already built more advanced routines, adapting your strategy for long-term success is key to keeping your body strong, lean, and energized.

---

1. Adapting the 15-Minute Plan for Long-Term Use

The 15-minute workout plan has been a cornerstone of your fitness journey so far, offering quick and effective routines that fit seamlessly into your schedule. However, as you continue to make progress, it's essential to evolve this plan to ensure long-term sustainability.

Benefits of Keeping a Short Workout Routine:

- **Time-Efficient:** The beauty of a short, 15-minute routine is that it's accessible, even on your busiest days.
- **Consistency:** Shorter workouts make it easier to stay consistent without feeling overwhelmed or burned out.
- **Adaptable:** As your fitness level increases, these sessions can be modified for greater intensity without sacrificing time.

Making It Sustainable:

- **Increase Intensity Gradually:** As you build strength and endurance, consider increasing the intensity of your workouts by adding resistance, increasing reps, or using heavier weights.
- **Add Progressions:** Instead of just repeating the same moves, progress to more complex versions of the exercises to challenge your body in new ways.
- **Schedule Rest and Recovery:** Incorporate active recovery days into your weekly routine to prevent burnout and give your muscles time to repair and grow.

---

2. Adding Variety to Workouts to Prevent Boredom

One of the biggest challenges with any long-term workout routine is preventing boredom. When you do the same exercises repeatedly, you might lose motivation and enthusiasm. To keep your workouts engaging and challenging, here's how you can add variety.

Ways to Spice Up Your Core Routine:

- **Alternate Between Cardio and Strength:** Mix high-intensity cardio sessions with core-focused strength training. This combination maximizes fat burning while toning your abs.
- **Try Different Formats:** Alternate between circuit training, supersets, or interval training for a fun and challenging twist.
- **Experiment with Equipment:** Incorporate resistance bands, dumbbells, medicine balls, or stability balls into your workouts. These tools can add variety and new challenges for your core muscles.
- **Change the Environment:** Take your workouts outdoors or to the gym. A change of scenery can keep things fresh and motivating.

Sample Variety Workouts:

- **Core Strength & Cardio Blast:** Perform a circuit alternating between 30 seconds of cardio (e.g., jumping jacks) and 30 seconds of core exercises (e.g., Russian twists).
- **Strength Training Circuit:** Mix core moves with full-body strength exercises like

squats, lunges, or push-ups to work on overall fitness.

- **Functional Training:** Add real-life movements, like kettlebell swings or woodchops, to train your core for everyday activities and sports.

---

3. Incorporating Functional Training for Overall Fitness

Functional training is about improving movements that you perform daily, such as bending, lifting, twisting, and reaching. By adding functional exercises to your routine, you not only maintain a flat belly but also enhance your overall fitness and mobility.

Why Functional Training Matters:

- **Prevents Injury:** It helps your body build strength in ways that reduce the risk of injury during everyday activities.
- **Increases Core Stability:** Functional exercises often engage multiple muscle groups, improving core stability and strength for real-life movements.
- **Boosts Functional Strength:** These exercises train your muscles to work together more effectively, improving performance in daily tasks.

Functional Training Movements for Core Health:

- **Kettlebell Swings:** Engages the entire body, especially the core, while enhancing power and flexibility.
- **Medicine Ball Twists:** A rotational move that targets the obliques and helps with spinal mobility.
- **Deadlifts:** Not only strengthens the core but also improves posture and engages the back and glutes.
- **Farmer's Carry:** Improves grip strength, core stability, and overall body control.

---

4. Long-Term Strategies for Maintaining Motivation

Staying motivated for the long haul is crucial to your success. It's easy to get caught up in the initial excitement of your transformation, but maintaining your fitness goals requires more intentional effort.

Tips for Staying Motivated:

- **Set New Challenges:** Continually set new fitness challenges to keep yourself engaged. Whether it's increasing your weight, reps, or the number of circuits, small milestones will keep you motivated.

- **Find a Workout Buddy:** Partnering with a friend or joining a fitness community can help you stay accountable and motivated.
- **Celebrate Small Wins:** Recognize progress, even if it's not directly related to fat loss. Celebrate strength gains, improved endurance, or better flexibility.
- **Track Your Progress:** Keep a fitness journal or use an app to log your workouts, meals, and progress. This can provide both insight and motivation to continue improving.

5. Conclusion: Embracing a Sustainable Fitness Lifestyle

Transitioning to a sustainable routine is about finding balance. By adapting your 15-minute plan, incorporating variety, and focusing on functional training, you'll not only maintain your flat belly but also improve your overall fitness and quality of life.

The key to long-term success is consistency, variety, and listening to your body. Keep challenging yourself, adapt your routine as needed, and celebrate every victory—no matter how small. Your fitness journey doesn't end here; it's about creating lasting habits that enhance your well-being and strength for years to come.

Chapter 15: Advanced Challenges

As you continue on your fitness journey and your body adapts to your routine, it's essential to challenge yourself in new ways to avoid plateaus and keep progressing. In this chapter, we'll dive into advanced techniques to take your workouts to the next level. By adding weights or resistance, and increasing the intensity and duration of your core workouts, you can build even more muscle, burn more fat, and develop a leaner, stronger core. Let's explore how to incorporate these advanced challenges into your training for maximum results.

---

1. Adding Weights or Resistance to Workouts

Incorporating weights or resistance into your core workouts is an effective way to increase strength and muscle definition. Not only does it intensify the exercise, but it also recruits more muscle fibers, improving endurance and muscle tone. Here's how to safely and effectively add resistance to your core training.

Benefits of Resistance in Core Workouts:

- **Muscle Growth:** By adding resistance, your muscles are forced to work harder, which leads to greater muscle growth and definition.

- **Increased Calorie Burn:** Resistance exercises require more energy, meaning they help you burn more calories during and after the workout.
- **Enhanced Stability:** Weights challenge your core in new ways, improving overall body stability and balance.

Types of Resistance for Core Workouts:

- **Dumbbells or Kettlebells:** Use these for exercises like Russian twists, side bends, or weighted crunches. By holding a dumbbell or kettlebell during these movements, you'll activate more muscle fibers in the core.
- **Resistance Bands:** Resistance bands are great for adding resistance to exercises like leg raises, bicycle crunches, or plank variations. They provide a consistent level of resistance and can be adjusted for difficulty.
- **Medicine Balls:** These are perfect for rotational movements or slam exercises. Medicine balls add dynamic movement to exercises like overhead slams, wall balls, or rotational throws, giving you both strength and cardiovascular benefits.
- **Weighted Vests:** Wearing a weighted vest while performing bodyweight exercises like planks, push-ups, or sit-ups increases the resistance without requiring additional equipment. It can help boost intensity and build endurance.

Example Resistance Exercises:

- **Weighted Russian Twists:** Sit with your knees bent, holding a dumbbell or kettlebell with both hands. Lean back slightly, engage your core, and twist your torso from side to side, tapping the weight to the ground next to your hip each time.
- **Dumbbell Side Bends:** Stand tall with a dumbbell in one hand. Slowly lean to the side, bringing the dumbbell down toward your knee, then return to standing. Repeat on the other side.
- **Kettlebell Swings:** Holding a kettlebell with both hands, hinge at your hips, swing the kettlebell between your legs, and then explosively drive your hips forward to bring the kettlebell up to chest height. This movement targets the entire core and glutes.

---

2. Increasing Intensity and Duration as Fitness Improves

Once you've become comfortable with your core routine, the next step is to increase both the intensity and duration of your workouts. Progressively challenging yourself ensures that your body continues to adapt and improves your overall fitness level.

Ways to Increase Intensity:

- **Increase Reps or Sets:** If you're performing core exercises for 30 seconds, aim to increase the duration by 10-15 seconds as your fitness improves. Similarly, you can increase the number of sets you perform for each exercise.
- **Add Plyometric Movements:** Plyometrics, such as jump squats, jumping jacks, or plank jacks, add an explosive component to your workout, increasing intensity and improving cardiovascular health.
- **Faster Tempos:** Speeding up your reps or switching to faster tempos will increase the intensity of your exercises, forcing your muscles to adapt to a higher workload.
- **Circuit Training:** Perform a circuit of exercises without resting between sets. For example, move from Russian twists into planks, then hanging leg raises, and finish with a cardio burst like high knees or jumping jacks. This keeps the heart rate elevated, burns more calories, and enhances core strength.

Example Advanced Core Workouts:

- **Core Circuit:**
  - **Burpees with Push-Up:** 10 reps
  - **Russian Twists (weighted):** 20 reps per side
  - **Hanging Leg Raises:** 12 reps
  - **Rest 30 seconds and repeat for 4-5 rounds.**

This high-intensity circuit targets multiple muscle groups while giving your core an intense challenge.

- **Plyometric Core Workout:**
  - **Jumping Plank Jacks:** 30 seconds
  - **Mountain Climbers:** 30 seconds
  - **V-Sits (with leg extension):** 30 seconds
  - **Plank-to-Push-Up:** 30 seconds
  - **Rest for 1 minute, then repeat for 3-4 rounds.**

Ways to Increase Duration:

- **Add Extra Rounds:** If you've been doing 3 rounds of a core workout, try increasing it to 4 or 5 rounds to give your muscles more time under tension and push your limits further.
- **Longer Work Intervals:** Shift from a 30-second work/30-second rest format to a 40-second work/20-second rest format for increased intensity.
- **Full-Body Integration:** Instead of solely focusing on core exercises, add full-body movements like squats, lunges, and push-ups into your core routine. This ensures that your muscles are being engaged for longer periods, further increasing both fat burn and endurance.

3. Monitoring Your Progress and Staying Challenged

As you incorporate these advanced challenges into your routine, it's important to track your progress to stay motivated and ensure that you are continually improving. Whether it's through increasing weight, reps, or intensity, maintaining a record of your achievements will keep you focused on your goals.

Tracking Your Progress:

- **Keep a Workout Journal:** Record the weights used, the number of reps and sets performed, and the intensity level of each workout. This will help you identify areas of improvement and allow you to celebrate small victories.
- **Use Fitness Apps:** Many apps allow you to track your workouts and progress over time. Some even give you personalized suggestions for increasing intensity based on your past workouts.
- **Take Progress Photos:** Visually tracking changes in your physique is a great way to see how your body has transformed over time. These photos can serve as a powerful reminder of how far you've come.

Staying Challenged:

- **Set New Goals Regularly:** Once you meet one goal, set another. Whether it's increasing your plank hold time, adding a new exercise, or improving your speed, fresh goals will keep you focused.

- **Change It Up:** Every few weeks, switch your routine by altering exercises, sets, or intensity. This will prevent your workouts from becoming stale and keep your body adapting.

Chapter 16: Community and Support

Building a strong, lean core isn't just about the workouts and the nutrition—it's also about surrounding yourself with a supportive network that motivates you to keep going, shares valuable insights, and holds you accountable. In this chapter, we will explore the role of community in your fitness journey, how joining fitness groups can elevate your progress, and the importance of connecting with like-minded individuals who are working toward similar goals.

1. Joining Fitness Communities for Accountability

Fitness communities provide much more than just workout tips or encouragement—they offer a sense of belonging and accountability. Whether online or in person, these groups foster an environment where individuals can share their goals, celebrate successes, and face challenges together. Here's why joining a fitness community can significantly enhance your core-strengthening journey:

The Power of Accountability:

- **Motivation to Stick to Your Goals:** Having a community of people who are actively working toward similar goals can push you to stay consistent, especially on days when your motivation may be lacking. Accountability partners or group challenges can help you stay on track, ensuring you make steady progress.

- **Support During Tough Times:** Everyone faces setbacks, whether it's an injury, a busy week, or a loss of motivation. A fitness community offers support during these times, helping you bounce back quicker by providing emotional and practical encouragement.
- **Goal Tracking and Celebrating Milestones:** Communities provide a platform to set, track, and celebrate progress. Sharing milestones like a new personal best, hitting a fitness goal, or achieving a breakthrough with core strength can boost your morale and inspire others to keep going.

Types of Fitness Communities:

- **In-Person Fitness Groups:** These could be local workout classes, boot camps, or sports teams that you join to get involved in a structured, supportive environment. Being able to meet face-to-face with others who are on the same fitness journey can create a sense of camaraderie.
- **Online Communities:** Social media platforms like Facebook, Instagram, and Reddit offer countless fitness groups where people share advice, progress photos, and their experiences. Online forums and apps (e.g., MyFitnessPal, Strava, or Fitbit) also provide spaces for users to track their

workouts, ask questions, and stay motivated.

- **Fitness Challenges:** Participating in online or local fitness challenges (such as 30-day core challenges) provides a structured plan for consistent improvement. These challenges foster competition and friendly rivalry, which can push you to perform at your best.
- **One-on-One Accountability Partners:** If you prefer more personalized support, finding an accountability partner who shares your fitness goals can be incredibly effective. Whether it's a friend, a workout buddy, or a coach, having someone to check in with regularly increases your chances of success.

How to Get the Most Out of Fitness Communities:

- **Engage Regularly:** Actively participate in the community by commenting, sharing your progress, and responding to others. The more involved you are, the more you'll benefit from the support.
- **Ask Questions:** Don't be afraid to reach out with questions or ask for advice. Most fitness communities are filled with experienced members who are happy to share their knowledge.
- **Give Back:** Offer support to others who may be struggling or looking for tips. The more you contribute, the more you'll feel

part of the group and gain valuable insights from others.

2. Sharing Progress and Challenges with Like-Minded Individuals

One of the most rewarding aspects of being part of a fitness community is the ability to share both your progress and your challenges. Not only does this help you stay motivated, but it also provides you with valuable feedback and advice from others who understand exactly what you're going through.

The Importance of Sharing Progress:

- **Inspiration for Others:** When you share your successes, no matter how big or small, you inspire others to push through their own challenges. Whether it's mastering a new core exercise, achieving a fitness milestone, or reaching a personal best, your progress can serve as a reminder to others that success is possible with persistence and dedication.
- **Tracking Progress with Others:** Sharing progress photos, workout logs, or fitness milestones in a community creates a sense of collective growth. As you document your transformation, you not only hold yourself accountable but also celebrate the achievements of others.

- **Constructive Feedback:** Posting your progress—whether it's a new move you've learned or an increase in strength—often invites constructive feedback. Someone in your community may have tips or modifications that will help you reach your goals faster and more safely.

Facing and Sharing Challenges:

- **Support Through Plateaus:** Every fitness journey faces obstacles, and it's important to acknowledge when things aren't going as planned. By sharing your struggles—whether it's difficulty hitting a certain rep count or feeling frustrated by a lack of visible progress—you can receive feedback, suggestions, and encouragement from the community to help you break through those plateaus.
- **Emotional Support:** Fitness journeys often come with emotional highs and lows. Sharing the emotional challenges of staying motivated, overcoming self-doubt, or dealing with personal obstacles can help you receive the support you need to stay focused on your goals.
- **Problem-Solving Together:** Fitness communities are great places to brainstorm solutions to obstacles. Whether it's dealing with a nagging injury, finding time to work out, or figuring out how to overcome lack of energy, these groups can provide creative

solutions and ideas you may not have considered.

How to Share Effectively:

- **Be Honest:** Share your progress and challenges openly and honestly. The more real and authentic you are, the more likely you are to receive meaningful support and encouragement.
- **Use Photos and Updates:** Progress photos, workout videos, or updates on your achievements can add a personal touch to your posts and help others track your journey. These can also help you visually see the progress you've made, which can be incredibly motivating.
- **Celebrate Together:** Don't forget to celebrate the wins, both big and small! When you hit a milestone or achieve a goal, share it with your community. The support you'll receive will make the accomplishment even more rewarding.

---

3. How Community Helps Overcome Challenges

While individual motivation is crucial, community support can be a game-changer when it comes to overcoming fitness challenges. Whether you're dealing with the pressure of self-doubt, injuries, lack of time, or struggling with consistency, a fitness community can offer solutions and solidarity that might not come from working out alone.

Dealing with Setbacks:

- **Support During Injuries:** If you're recovering from an injury, being part of a fitness community helps you stay positive and on track. Community members who've gone through similar experiences can offer advice on safe recovery exercises, stretching, and how to adjust your routine while healing.
- **Overcoming Time Constraints:** Many people struggle with finding time to work out, but sharing your scheduling issues with a fitness community can help you find new solutions. Fellow members can share time-saving tips, quick workout routines, and strategies for incorporating fitness into a busy lifestyle.
- **Boosting Consistency:** A strong community helps you maintain consistency, especially on days when motivation is low. Whether it's a weekly check-in, workout challenges, or group workouts, these structures can help you stick to your routine and make fitness a habit.

Building Long-Lasting Relationships:

Fitness communities don't just help you stay motivated; they also foster meaningful relationships. Sharing your journey with others, facing challenges together, and celebrating victories builds trust and camaraderie. These relationships often extend beyond fitness and can lead to long-term friendships and support systems that last far beyond your initial goals.

The Strength of Community

Fitness is never a solo journey—having the right support network can transform your experience and propel you to new heights. Fitness communities not only provide accountability but also offer valuable insights, encouragement, and a sense of belonging that can make your goals feel more attainable. By sharing both your progress and challenges, you'll stay motivated, overcome obstacles, and make lasting connections with others who share your passion for fitness. Whether online or in person, the power of community is a key element in achieving and maintaining a flat, strong core.

Conclusion: Your Flat Belly Fix

Achieving a flat belly and maintaining it is a journey, not a destination. It's about more than just the physical results—it's about the mindset, the consistency, and the commitment to taking care of your body in a way that nurtures its strength, energy, and overall health. As you finish this guide, remember that your journey is unique, and every step you take is a victory in itself.

Celebrate Progress, No Matter How Small

One of the most important lessons to embrace on your fitness journey is the value of celebrating every single bit of progress, no matter how small it may seem. Whether it's losing a few inches around your waist, feeling more energized after a workout, mastering a new exercise, or simply sticking to your routine, these milestones matter. Each success brings you closer to your goal, and every small step contributes to a bigger transformation.

Sometimes, the journey can feel slow, and results might not appear overnight, but remember that lasting changes come from consistent efforts. Celebrate the fact that you're making healthier choices, taking time for yourself, and investing in your wellbeing. It's all part of the process, and it all counts.

The Importance of Consistency and Balance in Achieving Fitness Goals

Consistency is the secret to success. It's not about perfection, but about staying committed to your goals, even when things get tough. Regular exercise, balanced nutrition, and mindfulness about your body's needs will always outweigh the occasional indulgence or missed workout. Life can be unpredictable, but building healthy habits and sticking to them—one workout, one meal, one mindful moment at a time—is what leads to long-term success.

Balance is just as important. It's easy to focus on one area, like your core, and forget that true health is built on a foundation of overall wellness. Core workouts are essential, but they should be complemented by full-body strength training, cardiovascular health, proper nutrition, and recovery strategies. Equally, as you progress, remember that it's not just about looking good but feeling great. Strive for a balance of strength, flexibility, energy, and mental clarity to achieve your best version of health.

A Final Motivational Note to Embrace Your Journey

Your journey toward a flatter belly and a stronger core is not just about the physical appearance—it's about creating a lifestyle that promotes health, confidence, and vitality. By incorporating the principles shared in this book—effective workouts, balanced nutrition, mindfulness, and recovery—you're on the path to not just achieving your fitness goals, but sustaining them long-term.

Embrace the process and enjoy the small victories along the way. Know that there will be challenges and setbacks, but they don't define you—they're simply part of your growth. In those moments, remember why you started and how far you've come. Every challenge you overcome makes you stronger, more resilient, and even more committed to living a healthy and balanced life.

So, whether you're starting with a 15-minute routine or taking your training to the next level, take pride in the commitment you're making to yourself. Your flat belly fix is not about perfection, but about embracing consistency, balance, and the journey itself. Keep moving forward, and know that your body—and your mind—are capable of amazing things.

Your journey toward a flatter belly is just the beginning of a healthier, more empowered you. Stay focused, stay positive, and never forget to celebrate your progress. Keep going, and keep believing in yourself—because the best is yet to come.

www.ingramcontent.com/pod-product-compliance
Lightning Source LLC
Chambersburg PA
CBHW071027250726
48653CB00005B/1749